THE GRATEFUL HEART

Diary of a Heart Transplant

Candace's Story

Candace Moose lives in Huntington, New York, on the North Shore of Long Island. She received immunizations in August 2001 in anticipation of traveling to Malawi, Africa, to help children suffering from AIDS. Soon after the shots she fell prey to an extraordinarily rare and generally fatal disease known as giant cell myocarditis. She received a heart transplant that October, and fought bravely and successfully to survive many obstacles in her recovery. She received caring help from many hands as she healed – from doctors, nurses, and other medical staff as well as family, church, and friends near and far.

This book is an expression of her faith and gratefulness. – *Editor*

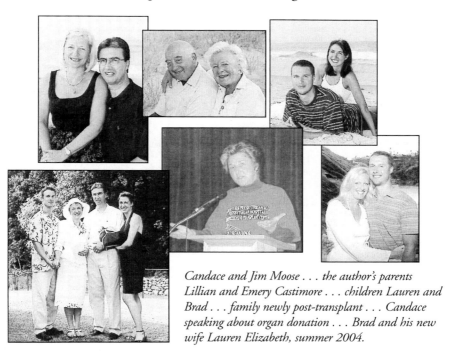

Candace and Jim Moose . . . the author's parents Lillian and Emery Castimore . . . children Lauren and Brad . . . family newly post-transplant . . . Candace speaking about organ donation . . . Brad and his new wife Lauren Elizabeth, summer 2004.

To my editor, Terry Walton,
without whose love, encouragement and skill
this book would never have come to be.

THE GRATEFUL HEART

Diary of a Heart Transplant

♥

"For out of the abundance of the heart, the mouth speaks."

– Matthew 12:34

Candace C. Moose

Every effort has been made to recall events
and attribute language with accuracy.
The author will be happy to correct mistakes or
errors of understanding in future editions.

❤

©2005 Candace C. Moose
Rosalie Ink Publications ▪ PO Box 291 ▪ Cold Spring Harbor, NY 11724 ▪ RosalieInk.com
First Edition ▪ All rights reserved
Editing & Production by Terry Walton ▪ Design by Inger Gibb
Printed in the U.S.A.
Library of Congress Control Number: 2004118150 ▪ ISBN 0-9711869-2-8

Dedication

I'd like to dedicate this book to my family and friends who stood by me throughout the darkest hours of my life. To my family, my wonderful husband Jim, my children Brad and Lauren, my parents, my sister Mary Ann, my brother Sam, his wife Joan and his children Matt and Robin, and my cousin Jan Tanis Jorritsma and her mother, my aunt, Rose Tanis, and the entire Moose clan, I love you more than words can say. To this day, I am not sure who suffered the most during the fifty-three days of my hospitalization – all of you or me. Additionally, to our dear, dear friends Anne and Bill Gray, Patti and Rich Redline, Ron and Helen Harris, the Poettgen family, our neighbor Pat Wagner, Bill and Carol Benner, Ida Carpenter, my former boss Diana Wilson, my grammar school friends Gary Schagelin (deceased), Betty DePue, Deborah Kishbaugh, and Joy Shue and the teaching staff of Bloomsburg school, thank you for your unfailing support.

I dedicate this book as well to the pastors and the congregations of churches that not only nurtured my faith through the years, but also steadfastly supported me and my family throughout my illness. God's light and love so clearly shined through the cards sent, the deeds done and the prayers offered by so many wonderful people. We as a family surely felt supported and cared for by the many acts of kindness.

Thank you – To Rev. and Mrs. Carl Luthman, formerly of the Lafayette Federated Church in Lafayette, New Jersey, where I spent some of the happiest days of my youth, where I was confirmed and married and our first child was baptized. To Rev. and Mrs. William Bender, formerly of Lower Valley Presbyterian Church in Califon, New Jersey, where Jim and I raised our children with the support and friendship of Cynthia Woerner and Susan Huntington. To Rev. Drew Byers, current pastor of the First Presbyterian Church of Newton, New Jersey, my grandparents' church where my parents were married and where we worshiped during the years that we lived on the farm with our children. To Rev. and Mrs. Craig Williams of Trabuco Canyon Presbyterian Church in Trabuco Canyon, California, our dear friends. This is where Jim and I learned how to be adults without children living at home, participated in building a new church and in the meantime formed a deep and abiding friendship with the pastor, his wife Dee and our Covenant Group partners Don and Ann Schulze. One thing I've learned from this experience is that you never really leave a church when you move from one part of the country to another. You simply take the congregations with you in your heart as you remain in theirs.

. . . To the Revs. David Bowman (deceased), Charles Cary, former Interim Pastor, and Regina Kokontis, former Associate Pastor of Old First Presbyterian Church in Huntington, New York, where in my retirement I was looking for a new direction for my life in mission work and found pastoral care and unrelenting support. To my friends in that congregation who have borne the burden of my care through countless acts of kindness joined with grace, my special thanks to Rizz Dean, my mentor, Mike Hawryluk, for sharing Kathleen, my confidante, my friend and my chauffeur on many 6 a.m. trips to Manhattan's NewYork-Presbyterian Hospital/Columbia, Judy Lee, Sandy Lange, Betty Fraser, Eloise Shakeshaft and so many others.

. . . To the Rev. Robert Schuler of the Hour of Power and the Rev. Charles Stanley of In Touch Ministries, who through their television ministries provided me and I am sure many others with the Sunday worship experience and spiritual enrichment for months following my surgery when I was homebound.

And beyond all I thank the health care professionals who cared for me throughout this ordeal. My undying affection and admiration belong to Dr. Mario Deng, heart failure and post-transplant physician. Dr. Deng, you affirm the life in me, which gives me the courage to keep on fighting. I am truly grateful to Dr. Leslie Cooper of the Mayo Clinic, who consulted on my case at the invitation of Dr. Deng, and who is the nation's leading researcher in giant cell myocarditis.

To the doctors, nurses, medical professionals and support staff of Huntington Hospital, specifically Dr. Charles Mascioli and Dr. David Sacknoff, and from St.

Francis Hospital in Roslyn, Dr. Alan Goldman, Dr. Steven Greenberg and Sister Katherine Murphy, and especially to everyone at NewYork-Presbyterian Hospital/Columbia in Manhattan – you will always be in my heart. To Dr. Ulrich Jorde, Dr. David Smull, Dr. James Coromilas, Dr. Yoshifumi Naka, Dr. Deborah Davis Ascheim, Dr. Sean Pinney, Dr. Matthew Maurer, the nurses and staff of the Heart Transplant Clinic, especially Sue Cech and Denise Groff, Mary Singh, JoAnn Padula, Elizabeth Burke, Sue Schnell, Cynthia Fox and Kim Hammond. To the entire Critical Coronary Care Nursing Staff, especially Remy Cordeta, Susan Sicat, and Jessie Castneda, and on 7 Hudson North, especially Paquita Maitem, and on 7 Hudson South, especially Aida Constancio, Sylvia Francis, Jennifer Cooper, Brian Salazar, Nelson Mendoza, Alicia Alleyne. To the Transplant Critical Care Unit Staff, especially Oliver Diaz, and the Cardiac Transplant Social Workers, especially Marni Alexander, Anne Lawler, and others whose names I cannot remember from those challenging days, thank you with all my heart for your love and your care.

And finally, heartfelt thanks to the health professionals who cared for me at home. To my physical therapist Jim Lewandowski, who pushed me, encouraged me and humored me throughout a long and difficult recovery. To my homecare chemo and IV nurses, especially Linda Bel, who made an extremely unpleasant procedure less so through her obvious love and caring. To Ruth Riley, my Complex Case Manager from Empire Blue Cross and Blue Shield, for her humanity, dedication and understanding in holding our hands through the insurance process. And last but not least to Geraldine Warren, Director of Volunteers for the New York Organ Donor Network, for listening and caring.

I would ask that you remember the following people in your prayers as you read this book: the families who in their time of most profound grief find it in their hearts to donate their loved ones' organs, as well as the people on waiting lists for donor organs, the people dying of AIDS in many parts of Africa and in other parts of the world, the children of the victims of AIDS who are and will be left as orphans if we don't do something now.

God bless the life in you all. CM

Complementary Worlds:
A Doctor's Perspective

This book is a unique experience for me to read because I am Candace Moose's transplantation cardiologist.

All the moments of suffering, of despair, and of hope that she describes from her own perspective, and from those of her husband and children, I remember very well from my perspective.

On one side, we remember the same situation. On the other, these same situations represent completely different worlds of experiences. The unique thing is that these worlds – in an irreducible way complementary – viewed alongside each other represent the process that Candace Moose and her family went through . . . from a shocking life-threatening event to a perspective of hope.

To have provided insight into these interconnected perceptions of suffering and healing, with the underlying units of patient, family and health care team viewed conceptually together, is the lasting achievement of Candace Moose's book – from my perspective.

– *Mario C. Deng, M.D.*
  Director of Cardiac Transplantation Research
  Columbia University Department of Medicine, Division of Cardiology
  New York-Presbyterian Hospital/Columbia

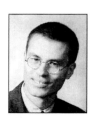

Contents

Timeline –
August 17, 2001, to the Present

2001

August 17 – Immunizations for trip to Malawi, Africa

August 24 – First hospitalization – Huntington, then transfer to St. Francis

August 27 – Cardioverter-defibrillator implanted

September 3 – Discharged from St. Francis Hospital

September 4 – Ambulance to Huntington Hospital Emergency Room

September 5 – Transferred to New York-Presbyterian Hospital/Columbia

September 29 – Placed 1A on United Network of Organ Sharing transplant list

October 1 – Transplant surgery; discharged October 11

October 11-November 24 – Six-week stay with parents

October 16 – Readmitted for rejection; discharged October 20

2002

June – 2nd major rejection; at-home treatment

July – Pacemaker inserted

October – Car accident

November – Stroke

December – Defibrillator inserted

2003

January-December – Healing time

2004

January-September – Healing time

October – Anniversary: three years post-transplant

Foreword
– A Husband's Perspective

"Who can find a virtuous wife? For her worth is far above rubies. The heart of her husband safely trusts her. Strength and honor are her clothing; she shall rejoice in time to come. She opens her mouth with wisdom, and on her tongue is the law of kindness." – Proverbs 31:10, 11, 25, 26

The story you are about to read is being told by Candace herself, although it could just as easily have been told by Brad and Lauren, our children, or by me. The details and the perspective would differ, of course, according to the storyteller, but the theme would be the same. Brad would convey the depth of his sorrow and the many levels of heartbreak and hopelessness he felt given both his mother's condition, and the weight of his concern for his sister – then living on the West Coast – having to deal with these tragic events. Lauren, just as insightful and intuitive as her mother, would convey the overwhelming feelings of loss as she watched her soul mate and the person she is closest to in the world slip away, while trying to comfort her family on the East Coast and manage her work in California. I would be tempted to describe, in great detail, the wonderful person I had married, and the grief that consumed me internally as I tried to mull my way through the pain of seeing her get weaker every day in the hospital, while I was still holding a job and trying to keep family and friends up to date on the unfolding events.

While the three of us would inevitably describe the story of seeing something terrible happening to Candace, as we watched like helpless bystanders, Candace herself writes from a completely different perspective. Candace's story is not about self-pity, but about faith and the happiness that comes with surviving the worst things one can imagine. It is a story about grace under pressure. We all know the facts, but she is the only one who can really tell the story – because it is about her response to the events, not merely the events themselves.

In the aftermath, it is clear to me that a person's true nature comes out during times of great adversity. I knew, perhaps as well as anyone, that Candace was a wonderful person. She has always been one of those people whose insight into, and interest in, others forms much of her personality. She is warm and outgoing, interested in everyone, quick to make friends, and always working to put people at ease. This type of behavior may be common at social events and cocktail parties, but is a little more difficult to pull off when you are in heart failure, in the worst pain of your life, and full of the anxiety that comes with not knowing whether you are going to live another day.

It was in these circumstances that Candace simply decided that focusing on her faith in God was the only chance she had of surviving the ordeal. And as a manifestation of that faith she decided she was going to be the best patient that the hospitals and staff had ever seen. To this end, she learned the name of every member of the medical staff, from doctors, to nurses, to nurses' aides, to IV technicians to x-ray staff to dieticians.

I was in her room one night shortly after she had been admitted to NewYork-Presbyterian Hospital/Columbia, when a team of medical professionals were trying to insert an arterial line into one of her ankles. Candace had a critically low blood pressure – which meant that no pulse was discernible as they began to cut into her ankle deeply enough to find an artery. They finished an hour later, after the ninth incision, without using an anesthetic agent, the deep arterial line finally in place. I went home that night and cried about both the pain she had to suffer and the courage and grace she had shown.

The story of her strength and bravery was repeated dozens of times during Candace's ordeal in the hospital, during the transplant, and during the extended recovery. She comforted the staff, the other patients, our children, our extended family, and me. During times of heart failure and pain, through the relentless progression of the disease killing her heart, and with the fear of not living long enough for a heart to become available, Candace would make certain to tell me to leave her room by a certain hour so that I could sleep and be rested to return the next day. Remarkable, thoughtful wife.

Candace continued her inspirational role during her recovery after the transplant, starting with her informal adoption of two young men who received heart transplants around the same time. Always encouraging both patients and families, she had a kind word for everyone. When she was well enough, on her return trips to the hospital after her discharge, she started baking for the staff, quickly zeroing in on the weakness of her post-transplant physician, Dr. Deng, for chocolate. She has become active in the New York Organ Donor Network and has been involved in several programs to raise awareness for organ donation. She had me save each of the hundreds of cards she received during her illness, and she has written thank-you notes to almost everyone.

While none of this surprises me in the least, I still find Candace's response to her ordeal amazing. She continues to be the optimistic partner she has always been, and spends much more time taking care of others than I could have imagined under the circumstances. She talks about feeling fortunate that she has had this experience, because it has made her a better person. We both have a new perspective about the little things in life we used to get upset about, and which we now tend to laugh about. I have learned to appreciate the woman I married even more, and I did not think that was possible.

The experience that Candace had to go through still makes me angry. Why did it happen? Why did she have to suffer so? Why could I not do more to ease her pain?

At the same time, though, it makes me appreciate Candace's strength. It makes me appreciate the incredible capabilities of modern medical science in general and of the staff of NewYork-Presbyterian Hospital/Columbia in particular. And it reminds me constantly that God watches over us and does indeed answer prayers. Candace's story is one that evokes every emotion, just like the life that we all sometimes take for granted.

– James A. Moose
Fall 2004

About Candace, From Three Friends

God's latest gift to me is the friendship of Candace Moose. The trips to the hospital and the seemingly endless routine of waiting gave us a wonderful opportunity to really get to know each other, to talk about serious matters as well as exchange recipes and to sometimes laugh together over silly things. Sharing the highs and lows, the joys and sometimes moments of almost despair in her determination to recover has immeasurably enriched my life. I feel as if I am the beneficiary in this relationship which came so close to never happening.

– Kathleen Hawryluk, Friend

When I first met Candace, I felt she was my alter-ego. We had so many local and world community interests in common, such as Union Theological Seminary and Save the Children. Then, when she became critically ill, she was an inspiration to us all. Her selflessness and optimism under the most trying of circumstances constantly amaze me. I have really done very little for her – the few times I drove her to the hospital, she was so upbeat, interested in others and obviously determined to overcome any setbacks, that I felt uplifted. Seeing how warmly she was greeted by all the staff at the hospital confirmed my belief that she was special.

– Rizz Dean, Friend

I am the newest of Candace's many friends, introduced by our shared acquaintance with Rizz Dean. What a blessing to be a new friend, ardent admirer, and editor honored to work on this remarkable book. It is written by a brave and truly delightful person, whom I have come to love.

– Terry Walton, Friend and Editor

Author's Preface –
Organ Donation . . . the Gift of Life

"Yet who knows whether you have come
to the kingdom for such a time as this?" – Esther 4:14

My story is not unique. Every transplant recipient has an equally dramatic story – one filled with drama, fear, despair, courage, patience and hope. We hear terrible news from our physician that we are failing, that we are going to die without a new organ. We wait and wonder if we will be one of the lucky ones to receive the life-saving gift. There is unbelievable joy at receiving the news that an organ has come for us. We know that now we have a chance to live. And finally, we struggle through a lengthy recovery, fighting every day to get just a little bit better. Through it all, we experience a profound sense of gratefulness to the donor family for their incredible gift. Concurrently, we feel immeasurable sadness for their loss.

In the midst of the crisis, on the line between life and death, we call upon every resource available to us to survive: a loving family, the support of friends, our faith and our innate will to live.

To me the highlight of my own story is the blessedly thoughtful involvement of the hospital personnel in my healing. Above and beyond the good decisions made regarding my medical care, came the many kindnesses giving me the courage to keep fighting, reinforcing my will to live. Without those gifts of grace I would not have survived. In this critical event in which everything you hold dear has been taken away from you – your health, your family, your freedom, your home, your dreams for the future – the medical professionals and support staffs of my three hospitals affirmed me as a person with dignity. I surrendered to their care and to God's keeping.

Curiously, of everything that happened, this is all that I remember. I don't remember every moment of the pain, every uncomfortable procedure or even

every critical event. But I believe I do remember every detail of the human inter-
actions with the medical staff, for they were my very lifeline.

What I remember so poignantly are these things: how safe I felt in Sister
Katherine's presence at my bedside, the kindness of the CCU nurses who lingered in my room when the chemotherapy was running, the understanding eyes
of the woman who swept my floor, the patience of the nurse who crayoned pictures with us in post-transplant recovery, the sacrifice of the PIC line nurse who
stayed at my bedside many long hours after his shift, the encouragement of the
physical therapist, the commitment and obvious caring of all of my heart failure
physicians as they battled my advancing disease, Dr. Deng's firm handshake that
seemed to communicate large doses of healing, the smile of my post-transplant
nurse whose job it was to teach me about all my medications before I went home,
the teasing of the x-ray technician, and last but certainly not least, the biopsy
room nurse Denise and her staff who still make me feel welcome, as if I were visiting old friends.

I live for all of these kindnesses. I live because of them. I accept each as a gift
from God, messages to make this crisis easier to bear.

Obviously, needing a new heart wasn't my first choice! I wanted simply to
be well. I wanted to be with my husband and my children. I wanted to
go home. I wanted life to return to normal. But in the absence of all
that, I was given two incredible gifts. The first was the heart that saved my life.
And embracing all this was the second gift – the staff, who gave me the gift of their
hearts. For both of these gifts I am eternally grateful.

My story happens to be told from my own Christian perspective. Yet kindness
and caring are transcendent values. I believe that many world religions share Judeo-
Christian values, that we all believe in the power of some omniscient, omnipotent,
almighty being that created goodness in all of us and who hears our prayers. My
book is a prayer of gratefulness for the gifts I received. My hope is that, no matter
what your belief system, you will find comfort, strength and even humor in my
story. And know that whether you are pastor or congregant, doctor or fellow patient,

friend or family member, you have the power to heal. Every word, every gesture, every act of kindness, however small, can strengthen someone who is ill.

Regarding the transplant experience specifically, no matter how difficult the journey we have traveled to become an organ recipient, we are the lucky ones . . . the ones who receive the organ and have the chance to live. Yet for the great majority of people on waiting lists, their story ends here. No organ comes in time.

Right now, today, no fewer than 85,000 Americans await a lifesaving transplant. Eight thousand of those live in the New York area. Tens of thousands more need tissue transplants. A new name is added to the national waiting list every thirteen minutes. A single donor can save up to eight lives through organ donation – and improve the quality of life of dozens of others through corneal, bone, skin and other tissue transplants. Seventeen men, women and children of all races and ethnic backgrounds die every single day for lack of a donated organ. Yet tragically, nationwide, half of the families asked about donation do not consent. Why? Mainly because they are unaware of their loved one's wishes, or they have misinformation about organ donation itself, or the critical need for this gift.

Please, make your wishes known to your loved ones. Remember the generous gift that saved my life. Sign a donor card, indicate your wishes on your driver's license and tell your family. (You might like to refer to the organ donor information attached here as Appendix A.) Registration means simply that in the event of your clinical death, your family will be approached and invited to help; surviving family must give consent before an organ can be considered for donation. And please don't assume that you are too old, or perhaps not eligible because you have a medical condition. Let the professionals decide. Or perhaps you are not comfortable with organ donation but would prefer just tissue or even a specific tissue, like a cornea, to be donated. Tell your family what you want. Make it clear. Write it down. It is the gift of life.

– Candace Moose, Heart Transplant 10/01/01
Fall 2004

♥

"In the midst of the crisis, on the line between life and death,
we call upon every resource available to us to survive: a loving family, the
support of friends, our faith and our innate will to live. . . ."

"Let us run with perseverance
the race that is set before us." – Hebrews 12:1

— ❤ —

1   THE CALL TO MY HEART

I was having the best summer of my life. Even better, I was having the best year of my life. I was on my way to Malawi, in southeastern Africa. On August 17, 2001, a sudden, catastrophic illness struck and changed the course of my life. For the next fifty-three days I was a patient in the critical care units of three different hospitals. The diagnosis, a rare and most often fatal autoimmune disease called giant cell myocarditis. As of that date there had been fewer than two hundred reported cases worldwide since 1905. What follows is a story about suffering and coming face to face with death. It is a real life story about the partnership of human frailty and human kindnesses and faith. It is a story about God's amazing grace.

February 2000

My husband, a pharmaceutical executive, decided to leave his job. This was of course a significant disruption in our lives. Though we are native to the East Coast, a previous job had brought us to California six years prior. We loved our home, our church, our neighborhood, our friends. In short, we loved our life there.

Jim would interview with several companies, three in California and one on the East Coast. At the time, my mother was desperately ill from the ravages of chemotherapy and radiation, treatment for non-Hodgkin's lymphoma. I wanted to come home nearer to New Jersey to care for her. Jim accepted a position with a firm on Long Island and would leave in May 2000. I would stay in California to complete arrangements for the move.

May 2000

We had done a corporate cross-country move once before. The drill is that Jim throws himself into his new job and the search for a new house while I handle my job and the selling of the old house. It means months of separation, not only of distance but also of time zones. Telephone calls have to be timed around work hours and within awake hours. Conversations are primarily about details, house repairs, buyer/seller demands, contracts, real estate issues and lawyers. There is little time or energy devoted to the marriage. It simply gets put on hold for the duration.

This was not the first time we had endured a long-term separation within our marriage. We had met on a blind date as sophomores in college and fallen madly in love. I stayed committed to my original plan of transferring to nursing school in Manhattan after sophomore year, as the college I was attending near Jim's university did not have a nursing program. We married in the summer after our junior year and went back to our separate schools, two hours apart, to complete our educations.

The second long-term separation had been years later in the fall of our youngest child's senior year of high school. Jim accepted the position with the company in California in October. Our son Brad was away at college, but it was not an opportune time for Lauren, our daughter, to transfer. She was in Advanced Placement classes, her college applications were in and she was signed up for scholastic tests. We decided as a family that Dad was ready for this challenge in his career and that Lauren and I would stay behind, sell the house and finish out her academic year and join him in June after graduation.

It was a very hard year for us all. We had vowed never to do it again, but alas, as life goes, the new Long Island position required that Jim leave again. I had responsibilities at my own job that I knew would take months to wrap up. By the time we got together, four months later, I would be exhausted.

Actually, I hadn't been feeling one-hundred percent for quite some time. Nothing specific, just fatigue. Quite simply, I worked too hard. I had been diagnosed with asthma in the prior year following bouts of bronchitis, which left me with permanent wheezing. After multiple exacerbations and several trips to the Emergency Room, I finally got on a preventive medication regime that brought the asthma under control. Asthma is an autoimmune disease characterized by hypersensitivity to an allergen in the environment. The medications given to treat the asthma events were not easy for me to tolerate. I have never tolerated medicine well, so I just never took it, with the exception of the occasional antibiotic. I've always had strange reactions to medications. If I took a pediatric dose of Tylenol or Advil, my husband knew I was really ill. When I told my physicians of the side effects I was having from the medications, they'd say there were no reports of similar side effects in the literature. Not very comforting. Were they implying that it was all in my head?

I had changed jobs just the preceding year in California, in the hopes of creating more balance in my life. The new job turned out to be even more demanding. When Jim left for Long Island I made the decision to retire with this move. My company was reluctant to let me go, so officially I took a leave of absence for three months to care for my mother.

By way of background, professionally I am a registered nurse. I had graduated from Cornell University–New York Hospital School of Nursing in 1973. Jim and I, as mentioned, were married while undergraduates. When I graduated, I was pregnant with Brad. My first job out of school was as a staff nurse in the Intensive Care Unit of a little community hospital in New Jersey where Jim had acquired his first pharmaceutical job. For the next several years, I worked part-time in the

Intensive Care Unit, the Critical Coronary Care and the Progressive Coronary units of the same hospital. Brad was born in February of 1974 and our daughter Lauren was born in November 1976. I worked part-time for the next couple of years. Hospital nursing continues to be a wonderful career for parents as you can work evening and night shifts and weekends around your family life.

Ultimately, I would leave clinical nursing in part because I had sores between my fingers that would not heal. In the critical care areas especially, nurses wash their hands, put on gloves, take off gloves and wash their hands again a thousand times a day. I thought the soaps were too harsh for my skin. I tried creams and ointments but to no avail. No one had ever heard of latex allergies in those days. No one yet knew that repeat exposure would leave nurses at particular risk for developing latex allergies years later.

My surprising "allergies" had in fact taken a dramatic turn years before when Lauren was just six months old. I went to the dentist for a routine filling of a cavity. The dentist gave me two boluses of Novocaine with Epinephrine in my lower jaw. I felt the needle enter the vessel. As an intravenous certified nurse, I could feel when the needle had penetrated the vessel wall. Novocaine is supposed to be injected into surface tissue, not vessels.

The dentist left the room to care for another patient, ostensibly to give the medication a chance to make my mouth numb. At first, I noticed that my visual field was narrowing. Then I realized I couldn't make my chest move to take in a breath. My nail beds turned black. I threw my torso against the metal tray to create a disturbance to attract the dentist's attention and then I passed out. When I came to, I was on the floor. My dentist's face was covered in perspiration, as though someone had poured a bucket of water over his head.

Looking back, I can't believe I dared to do this, or that the dentist let me do it, but I drove from the dentist's office one mile to my family physician. My doctor said that there had been no reported cases of allergic reactions to Novocaine. He said it was more likely that the two boluses of Epinephrine, which had been injected into a major vessel in my mouth, had put me into shock. The medical profession seldom uses the Epinephrine/Novocaine mix anymore. For the next twenty-five years I would have teeth filled, root canals performed and skin biopsies taken with no local anesthetic as I feared a similar reaction.

The dentist episode was my first code. In medical jargon, a sudden, unexpected near-death experience is a "code." From a clinical standpoint, it means that the heart has stopped providing oxygen to the major organs of the body such as the brain. Exactly as the literature describes, I traveled down a dark tunnel with a bright, warm light at the end. There was no fear, just a warm peaceful feeling. I knew I was not ready to go, that I wanted to live to raise my children. I woke up on the floor of the dentist's office. I had expected to wake up in heaven.

From that point on I would have a cardiac arrhythmia, or in laymen's terms an irregular heartbeat. With every menses, five days before onset, my heart would beat so erratically that it would prevent a night of sleep. The next day the arrhythmia would be gone. Over the years I would have several Holter monitor tests and echocardiograms to confirm that the condition was essentially benign and that treatment with anti-arrhythmic drugs was optional. The Holter monitor is a test that records an electrocardiogram over twenty-four hours. My results revealed multiple premature ventricular contractions, or extra beats, which due to their position in the beat-and-rest cycle of the ventricles, or large chambers of the heart, did not pose a threat to triggering a life-threatening arrhythmia. I chose not to be treated.

Back to the present. . . . We moved into our new home on the beautiful North Shore of Long Island in September of 2000. The movers put the furniture in the house and the boxes in the garage, and left. The house had less square footage and less storage space than the California house, so unpacking was no simple matter. I had to sort through the boxes, decide what we needed and what there was room for in the new house. I discovered boxes belonging to the children that hadn't been unpacked since the previous move. For the first time with a family move I wasn't trying to hold down a full-time job as well. I just resigned myself to the fact that unpacking would take months, and besides that, I was exhausted. To this day I haven't completely finished the task.

Now that we were settled in Long Island, my plan for retirement was to devote my life to doing something about the terrible pandemic of AIDS in so many of the countries in Africa. After almost thirty years in medicine and a career-long interest in AIDS, I felt I might have something to offer.

AIDS had emerged as a significant public health issue early on in my career, and, as the press reports, since its inception has killed more people than World War I, World War II, the Korean War, the Vietnam War and the Gulf War combined. It is the leading cause of death in sub-Saharan Africa and as we all know is rapidly becoming an epidemic in other parts of the world as well. The economic, social, political, health and ethical ramifications are profound, not only for the countries involved but also for all of us individually.

In sub-Saharan Africa, as newspapers remind us every day, AIDS has spread like wildfire – fueled by fear, ignorance, inaction, denial and isolation from the rest of the world. People with AIDS are ostracized from their society. Women and children are the most severely affected. Without any means of support they are left to die. In our own country – though behavioral changes have found only moderate success – with major advances in pharmaceutical science, the disease is still fatal but with treatment people do live longer. Yet with political instability, insurmountable debt and lack of political clout, as well as poverty and basic lack of medical infrastructure, most countries in Africa can offer only limited access to these medications. So a whole continent of people are dying at an alarming rate.

My own professional experience had prepared me well for the myriad issues surrounding AIDS. It had ranged from clinical practice in the hospital, to outpatient GYN medicine, to school nursing, to teaching and finally to monitoring investigational drug trials for pharmaceutical companies. AIDS affected the entire practice of medicine by changing how we think about body fluids. From the handling and receiving of blood products, to administering first aid to injured victims, to teaching prevention behaviors, to learning what chemicals kill the virus on work surfaces, the onset of AIDS in the early 80's changed medicine forever. Finally, after completion of my graduate degree (five years in night school!), had come the opportunity to work for a clinical research organization working on a large AIDS investigational drug trial. It was a wonderful experience. I was now doing exactly what I had longed to do.

Then, my husband accepted the pharmaceutical manufacturing position in California. I continued to work for the same company after the move, traveling and monitoring drug protocols in AIDS and other therapeutic areas, collecting data on side effects of the drugs, confirming that research sites had enrolled appropriate patients and verifying with site research staff that the drugs were being taken correctly.

By the time I reached my retirement as we returned to the East Coast in September 2000, I felt I had a unique perspective from which to view the disease from a variety of angles. More importantly, I felt as though God had been preparing me throughout my entire professional career for just this task. But for what exactly?

Since the move to Long Island I had begun researching both secular and religious organizations involved in AIDS projects in various areas of Africa. At the time, AIDS was receiving a lot of press. PBS ran an excellent series on the status of AIDS in sub-Saharan African countries. The United Nations convened a special session to address the issue worldwide. Congress pledged a small sum that activists described as a "criminal" amount of money to the UN AIDS Relief Fund. A rally in New York brought attention to the issue. The newspapers were filled with debate over pharmaceutical patent rights versus debt relief.

In the meantime, people were dying at an alarming rate, leaving millions of orphans behind. Press reports estimate that by the year 2010 there will be 44 million AIDS orphans in Africa – equaling the number of all elementary school children in the United States.

In the months after our move to Long Island I joined the Mission Committee of our local church in Huntington, to find out what the congregation was doing about AIDS in Africa. I talked to people in the church to let them know what I was interested in. When someone found an interesting article in *The New York Times* or a program on television on the subject they would let me know. They suggested names of people and organizations that I should contact.

June 2001

One of the women from my Bible Study group gave me information about a mission opportunity involving Africa. The project involved collecting bed sheets for hospitals in The Democratic Republic of the Congo and Malawi. In the hospitals where sheets are even available, I learned, patients receive one sheet at the time of admission. This is hard to imagine. Apparently, supplies are so critically short that patients are expected to return their one sheet, freshly laundered, at the time of discharge. Ours was thus a truly worthwhile project.

It was suggested that each church on Long Island pledge thirty sheets to help the national church meet its annual commitment to the African hospitals. The sheets had to be collected and delivered to a central shipping location by December 31, 2001. I asked other church members why we weren't involved in this project and the answer was that no one had volunteered to be chairman, so I volunteered. We pleged one hundred sheets!

I was so excited about my retirement. It afforded me the first opportunity in my life to really do mission work, even if only from a distance. Through the local Presbytery of Long Island office, I discovered that the Presbyterian Church USA also has an office adjacent to the United Nations in Manhattan, about thirty-five miles from my home. AIDS was a hot topic because of an upcoming international conference.

I contacted the Manhattan office and offered my volunteer services to help organize a workshop for spring 2002. The plan was to invite people working with AIDS patients in Africa to the PCUSA office near the United Nations, to discuss the issue and possible solutions. My first meeting at this office was scheduled for September 16, 2001. I wouldn't make it.

In June, my friend Rizz had invited me to an evening program sponsored by a group called Save the Children, as she knew they worked in Africa. They are a highly respected organization promoting the health and welfare of women and children, both in the US and around the world. The speaker was reporting on her group's recent trip to Nepal to visit projects funded by the organization. The purpose of the evening was to raise awareness about the needs of women and children of Nepal, and to raise money so that current programs could continue or expand and new programs could be started.

At the conclusion of the program, I asked a staff member if the organization was involved in AIDS projects anywhere in Africa. I explained my background and my desire to commit my retirement to this issue. The founder of the Long Island branch of the group overheard our conversation and interjected that not only did Save the Children have projects, but there was also a group going to Malawi in September and would I like to go along.

Truthfully, I had no intention of traveling to a third world country to visit AIDS projects and Malawi is one of the poorest. Malawi is a landlocked country in the southeastern section of the continent. It is slightly smaller than the state of Pennsylvania, I learned, and has a population of approximately ten million people. Over 800,000 Malawians are affected by HIV/AIDS. Life expectancy is a devastating thirty-seven years and annual per capita income is less than one thousand dollars. Poverty, disease, political unrest and lack of medical care are among the reasons Malawi is so troubled.

I am not an experienced international traveler. I couldn't imagine sitting still for a twenty-one-hour flight. And, I was scared to death to make the trip. I had been thinking more along the lines of working at Manhattan's PC/UN office and running projects stateside. I said I would give it serious consideration.

As it happened, Jim and I left on vacation with our grown children and my parents the next day. I never mentioned the trip to Malawi to anyone on the vacation or even when we returned home a week later. But the trip kept reappearing in my consciousness, in the mornings when I set aside time for meditation. God was tugging at my heart, but I was trying hard to resist. The coincidence of the sheet project from church and the trip with Save the Children was too profound to ignore.

I started to pray about it. There were three obstacles to my going: a minor health issue of mine just then that might require surgery, the travel – and the immunizations. I was nervous about the shots because of my odd reactions to so many things, but felt there should be no problem since statistically they are considered routine and safe.

July 2001

One by one, the obstacles disappeared. The minor health issue vanished with no surgery required. Next came the trip itself. Did I really want to travel that distance away from Jim, and place myself at risk of contracting a tropical disease or not have access to treatment for a severe asthma attack? Leave him to worry about me while trying to concentrate on his new position? And the third, the immunizations, seemed, as noted, statistically just fine.

I pondered all the issues. Jim did not want to risk losing me, but after much discussion of the pros and cons of the trip he pledged his support. It was an act of faith. I felt as though God was calling me to Malawi. I put my trust in Him.

I sent the following e-mail to a friend: "Africa is scary for all of those reasons and more. Political unrest, diseases, etc. I'm not a very experienced world traveler and I have no desire to be away from Jim. But right now, I want to go, see what I have to see, learn what I have to learn and come home safely. Please pray for me. I believe I am not a person of great courage. I guess I am about to find out."

In the meantime, with the Malawi trip still two months away, I was "having the best summer of my life." I had signed up for crewing classes through the local community summer recreation program. The program offered a series of six classes, each session lasting two weeks. By the time I got around to registering, only the last three sessions of the summer were open. I had intended to sign up for them all. . . .

The north coast of Long Island borders on Long Island Sound. The state of Connecticut is visible from the shoreline. The Sound is a popular site for sailing and powerboating. It is also exceedingly beautiful. The coastline is carved with many little inlets and coves, home to diverse species of wildlife, especially birds.

We live just a block from Huntington Bay, which empties into the Sound. On my daily walks with my dog I had seen the crew teams rowing just offshore. Having never lived so close to a body of salt water, I had never had the chance to row and I couldn't wait for classes to begin. I have always considered myself something of an athlete. My passion in life is tennis and I have always kept in shape by walking ten or fifteen miles a week. Rowing seemed the perfect thing.

The boathouse was within walking distance of my home, on the property of Coindre Hall – a former Gold Coast estate now deeded to the Town of Huntington. Classes began in mid-July. I had no idea that the sport demanded so much skill, strength and concentration. The boat holds nine people – eight crew and one coxswain who gives the rowing commands. The boat weighs two-hundred-fifty pounds and is twelve feet long – it takes nine people to lift the boat out of water, flip it over and carry it up on the dock to be washed and placed on a boathouse storage rack.

It's important that every member pay close attention and row in synchrony, I soon learned. If someone "catches a crab" or turns the oar blade the wrong way in the water when the boat is moving, the force of eight people rowing and moving the boat forward can flip the rower right out of the boat. Our first night out on the open water of the Sound, we rowed a mile out and a mile back. I was not the oldest participant, nor was I in the worst shape, but this is a very physically demanding sport and I loved every minute of it.

We rowed in the evenings at sunset. The light on the water, the warmth of the setting sun, the sight of birds, the gentle swell of the waves, the beauty of the clouds and the colors of the sunsets gave me a front row seat to the grandeur of God's creation. It was a deeply spiritual experience. I came home every night exhausted, dehydrated and exhilarated. I felt blessed that God had brought me to this part of the country so I could enjoy this incredible experience. I rowed for five of the six weeks, until the night before the immunizations.

August 2001

I sat down to do my daily devotions on the morning of August 16th. I use a devotional published by the Unity Church. The writings are always positive, and sometimes speak directly to whatever issue may weigh heavily on my spirit. That particular day, I remember, the study dealt with taking risks. The study suggested that one had to step outside of one's comfort zone and try something new. That God has given us many gifts that go untapped if we are not courageous enough to try new experiences.

That morning I felt as if God were speaking directly to me through this study. Following my devotions and prayers for friends and family, I sat alone in silence, allowing these minutes for just listening, waiting.

Meditation is not an easy exercise for me. A million thoughts try to force their way into my consciousness. But on that day, the silence deepened as it lengthened. I had the profound sense that God was present with me. It was what Anthony Bloom in his book *Beginning to Pray* would call a "silence with substance." I knew the encounter was significant; I just did not know why it had occurred. I left this morning time filled with an acute sense of the power, the love and the peace of God.

Months later, while at home recovering from the heart transplant on a Sunday morning, I was watching a television evangelist from Atlanta by the name of Charles Stanley of In Touch Ministries. He was preaching about finding inner peace. One of the steps he recommended was meditation. When we fill prayer time with declaring our concerns, he contended, we do not give God a chance to speak to us. He said that God could use the meditation as a time of preparation for a difficult time ahead. Little did I know what lay ahead after our encounter, God's and mine, on that morning of August 16th.

"We rowed in the evenings at sunset. The light on the water, the warmth of the setting sun, the sight of birds, the gentle swell of the waves, the beauty of the clouds and the colors of the sunsets gave me a front row seat to the grandeur of God's creation. It was a deeply spiritual experience. . . ."

"Father, all things are possible for You. Take this cup away
from Me; nevertheless, not what I will, but what You will." – Mark 14:36

2 THE BROKEN HEART

Friday, August 17, 2001

On the morning of Friday, August 17, I went to my physician to get the immunizations I needed to travel to Malawi. Several weeks before this visit I had asked my doctor if a person with my sensitivity to drugs could have both immunizations on the same day. He said there was no reason not to. The immunizations had to be given within six weeks of the travel date and we were scheduled to leave on September 29. The nurse asked if I would like her to review the potential side effects of the immunizations and I said no, I would let her know if I had a problem. I didn't want all the things that could possibly go wrong floating around in my head, lest I imagine them coming true.

As it happened, I had a luncheon scheduled with my new but dear friend Rizz following the Friday visit to the doctor. I had been introduced to her through a mutual friend from church who thought Rizz might be able to help me plug into organizations that needed volunteers. It turned out we had a great many shared interests and philosophies; Rizz took me under her wing and introduced me to organizations, people and places she thought I might be interested in and that could use my time and talents, including Save the Children.

We had a lovely luncheon, Rizz and I, at a special little restaurant called the Book Mark Café in nearby Oyster Bay. We talked about our children. I had the sense that blessedness was present at our meal and in our friendship, and felt grateful I was to be sitting there at that moment with this remarkable lady. Rizz has served in many leadership roles in her eventful lifetime. She still actively lobbies state lawmakers in Albany and visits local representatives to convey her opinion on impending legislation. Our shared membership at Old First Presbyterian Church in Huntington was the foundation, the common denominator of our friendship.

Sometime that Friday evening, eight hours or so after the immunizations, the tachyarrhythmia started – a rapid, irregular heartbeat (as noted in Glossary). It was after dinner and Jim and I were sitting on the couch watching television. I was aware that my heart was beating more forcefully than usual. At first I thought I was dizzy, but that wasn't it. The television screen kept moving. I realized that the force of my heartbeat was throwing my head slightly side to side. I had no pain, fever, sweating or discomfort of any kind in my jaw, chest or arms, other than the rapid and forceful irregular heartbeat. I thought this event was perhaps being triggered by my hormonal cycle, which was erratic as I was perimenopausal.

But on some level I knew this was different. This was the first time my heartbeat had been fast and irregular. Later as I lay in bed, the force of my heartbeat tossed my head a bit side to side on the pillow such that I could not sleep. I moved to one of the kids' bedrooms so I would not disturb Jim. As I lay there it felt as though my heart were beating out my back. I stayed awake most of the night. It never occurred to me to call the doctor and besides, it was Saturday and my doctor's offices were closed. This was certainly not an emergency. I surely know better now.

Sunday, August 19

Well, I had things to do and places to go. So despite my unease, I got through Saturday and on Sunday I drove to New Jersey. I offered to spend Monday scouting out possibilities for a new living situation for my son closer to his job. He had just finished graduate school and started a new job from which he could not ask for personal time to look for a new place. I did spend some looking around time, to no avail, but at least it was a good start. I was aware at night that my heartbeat was still irregular, but during the day there were more pressing matters and I forgot all about it.

That Monday evening I drove out to my parents' house one hour away in northern New Jersey. My dad was scheduled for surgery to repair an artificial knee joint Tuesday morning. He had to be at the hospital by 6 a.m. My mother was still recovering from the lingering effects of chemo and radiation for her non-Hodgkin's lymphoma and wasn't well enough to drive him anywhere at that hour. I volunteered to take him. We all joked and made nervous conversation. What a threesome we were. . . .

For the next two days I stayed at the hospital, either in the waiting room or at my father's bedside. As soon as I was confident he was out of danger and on the road to recovery, I headed home to Long Island. I still didn't feel well. I hadn't slept well, I was tired and I knew now that I needed to go to my doctor.

I got home Wednesday afternoon. When I called Thursday morning for an appointment, I was reminded that it was his day off.

Friday, August 24

Early Friday morning I took our dog Ruffie for a walk. As I climbed up the hill to our house, I realized I was winded. I thought it might be my asthma, but I wasn't wheezing. I took my asthma medication anyway but it didn't help. Jim offered to take me to the doctor or to the Emergency Room. I said no, that I was okay, and promised him I'd go directly to the doctor when he opened first thing this morning.

My local doctor's staff in Huntington said to come right in. When the doctor arrived to examine me, I told him about the tachyarrhythmia, the night sweats and that I really wasn't feeling well. I also told him the symptoms had started the day of the immunizations.

The nurse had already taken the electrocardiogram. The ECG revealed what he thought was a new "left bundle branch block" – reminiscent of a concern three months earlier – but they hadn't yet located my chart to compare it to the older version. I knew the earlier ECG had shown what I remembered was a "right bundle branch block": a conduction defect of the heart on the right side. Nothing much to worry about, we all agreed – the same old irregular heartbeat I'd had from time to time for years.

Normally as an electrical stimulus moves across the surface of the heart, which then causes the different parts of the heart to contract, it creates a pattern of waves that are recorded on paper with an electrocardiogram. The right side of the heart receives venous blood from the body and ejects it to the lungs for oxygenation. The left side of the heart receives the oxygenated blood from the lungs and ejects it into arteries, which carry fresh blood to the body. Physicians as a rule are more concerned with a conduction defect in the left side of the heart, as it may indicate a more critical event. Defects of the right side of the heart are more often associated with a chronic non-life-threatening condition.

As it turned out, my chart was still in the hands of my gynecologist who had wanted to speak to me directly about the results of an earlier appointment. The chart arrived before long and the doctor could now compare old and new ECG tracings. He came straight into the examining room and told me he believed I'd had a heart attack. I told him I didn't think so. He wanted me to go directly to the Huntington Hospital Emergency Room, right across the street, and be admitted to the Progressive Coronary Unit. He asked me to humor him. He said if my enzymes were normal, I could go home tomorrow. Cardiac enzymes are released into the bloodstream when there has been damage to the myocardial tissue, indicating in most instances an acute myocardial infarction – a heart attack. I asked if I could go home and pick up some things and make a few phone calls and he said, unequivocally, no.

In the Emergency Room I changed into a hospital gown, had some blood drawn and was placed on the cardiac monitor, and then waited for the room to become available. I called Jim at work. Three days earlier he had become CEO of a new company, spun off from the one he had come East to join. He was stunned by my news but not panicked. I was fairly cavalier, convinced I'd be going home the next day.

I was soon transported to the Progressive Coronary Unit, met the staff and got hooked up to a portable cardiac monitor and oriented to my new environs. Jim arrived shortly thereafter. I called my children, one in California and one in New Jersey, both at work, to tell them what was going on and not to worry, I was fine. Lauren told me later she was glad someone was finally paying attention to this irregular heartbeat, which she knew had been with me on and off for years. My husband was cracking jokes to the kids over the phone and the mood was light. I was after all just "humoring the doctor."

My doctor came into my room at about 4 p.m. He reported that the enzymes were in fact elevated and that I had had a heart attack. I was shocked. His plan was to move me within the next several minutes to the Coronary Intensive Care, where I would stay only until arrangements could be made to transfer me to St. Francis Hospital half an hour away in Roslyn, New York, that night. He explained that St. Francis specializes in heart diseases and would perform a cardiac catheterization to assess the status of my coronary vessels for blockage, and that they could perform angioplasty or bypass surgery immediately if necessary.

I stayed in CCU only long enough to get an intravenous line started, and to take a sedative. In the middle of that night EMT's, trained emergency medical professionals, transported me to St. Francis Hospital as planned. I overheard them commenting that my ECG looked an awful lot like ventricular tachycardia, a life-threatening arrhythmia. Sometimes there is disagreement between physicians in reading electrocardiograms. A bundle branch block causes the QRS complex (heartbeat waves) to widen on an ECG tracing, so a rapid BBB (bundle branch block of electrical impulses) looks a lot like V-tach (ventricular tachycardia). One of the rhythms is life threatening and the other is not. It's important although oftentimes difficult for the physician to make the distinction.

Saturday, August 25

I had arrived at St. Francis in the middle of the night on Friday. I was admitted to a semi-private room in a medical ward of the hospital. I sent Jim home with directions to call the kids in the morning and ask them to come. I was nervous about an electrophysiology study, planned to test the electrical function of my heart.

One of the cardiologists from the group responsible for my care came into my room at 3 a.m. to take my history and physical. He asked why I was there. I said I really didn't know, that my doctor said I had a heart attack, but that I didn't believe it. Denial is one of the classic reactions to this diagnosis. Per doctor's orders, the nurse started the standard acute myocardial infarction intravenous medications to dilate the coronary vessels and prevent further damage. She also started prepping me for cardiac catheterization, scheduled for first thing Saturday morning about four hours away. I signed the informed consent for the procedure. I think I slept.

A cardiac catheterization is performed by inserting a catheter into a vein, injecting dye and then taking pictures of the coronary vessels. I remember watching the fluoroscopy screen during the procedure. My coronary vessels looked like leafless trees against the background of a moonlit night. The cardiologist confirmed that I had no blockage.

I woke up in the Recovery Room, the only patient. I was attended by two nurses. One of them had just called the cardiologist to come back to the Recovery Room to take a look at my cardiac monitor. I was in a slow ventricular tachycardia, a life-threatening arrhythmia. They started medications to control the arrhythmia. I don't remember much of anything else about that day, except meeting a wonderful person named Sister Katherine.

Once stable, I learned later, I was moved to a six bed step-down unit. A step-down unit is for patients who need to be closely monitored but do not require critical care, but neither are they well enough to be put out on the general medical floor. The nurses on the day shift were warm, competent and caring individuals. The nurse/patient ratio in the unit is about one to three during the day. A curtain separates each patient's bed from the next. All beds are visible from the nurses' station, and each patient is only a step away from their reach. All patients in the room wore cardiac monitors enabling their cardiac rhythm to be visualized at the nurses' stations both in the step-down unit and out on the floor just outside the door.

Sister Katherine is the St. Francis Hospital clinical nurse specialist – her job is to improve nursing practice, and she is responsible for patient, staff and family education. She is one of those rare individuals who are perfectly suited to their job and secure in their own skin. She is both loved and respected by the staff she supervises and the patients she makes it a point to know. She had been through the unit several times each day over the weekend. It is her job not only to educate the staff but also to know which patients might present problems requiring her attention. It is her job to make sure there is adequate trained staff to handle any crisis. From her frequent visits I knew I was very much on her radar screen.

Sister Katherine introduced herself and we immediately connected; nurses have a common bond with other nurses, and I told her of my own professional CCU experience. I assume it's like war buddies who have served together in the military. You've both been in the trenches. You share a common history. Sister Katherine is a person of faith and so am I. Though a different faith, the difference was immaterial. She made a point of making me feel I was among welcome guests in her hospital. I was comfortable under her care. I felt safe on her watch.

Sunday, August 26

I was scheduled for the electrophysiology study the following morning, Sunday. My daughter had flown in from California, met at the airport by my husband. The cardiologist who performed the study had just come back from a family vacation in Israel the night before. He was relaxed and jovial, regaling the procedure room staff with stories about his trip.

I felt at first like a non-entity; a procedure rather than a person. The cardiologist didn't even address his remarks to me. Yet at the same time he behaved in such a confident manner that I came to feel I had nothing to be afraid of. Perhaps his casual conversation was intended to put me at ease, and after my initial sense of being ignored while I was trying so hard to cope with the feeling of my life being out of control, I did feel my fear subside.

I had read the educational materials about the procedure prior to signing the informed consent, and knew they hoped to find an aberrant site in the heart that was sending out an additional signal and causing my heart to beat irregularly. The aberrant site could then be ablated (cauterized with an electrical current), allowing the AV (atrial ventricular) node to take over as the natural pacemaker for the heart. But at the end of the procedure the cardiologist stated that no aberrant site could be found. Later, he told my husband that my heart was badly scarred and a defibrillator would be needed – a cookie-sized electronic device implanted just beneath the skin of the chest wall, with wires running to the heart. I woke up in my bed in the step-down unit where I had first met Sister Katherine.

The defibrillator surgery was all set for Monday. It was fairly standard and I was assured there was nothing to worry about. Lauren had reservations to return to California the next day, Brad would return to his job in New Jersey.

Monday, August 27

The kids were going to do some early morning grocery shopping for Jim and come to the hospital before my procedure. Jim himself would do chores around the house and come to the hospital later just ahead of the kids.

I was on the Operating Room schedule for 2 p.m. for the insertion of an ICD (implantable cardioverter-defibrillator). I met the implant doctor that morning. The device he had chosen had the capability to perform both cardioversion and defibrillation. Cardioversion is a low-voltage function of the pacemaker, which causes an electrical shock to be delivered to the heart to convert a rapid rhythm to a normal, slower rhythm. Defibrillation is a more powerful shock, which is delivered to a heart in the event of a non-life-sustaining rhythm called ventricular fibrillation.

Sometime that morning my heart stopped beating for the first time. The next thing I knew, Sister Katherine and many other people were standing around my bed. I felt as though I had been very far away, in a deep sleep. Sister Katherine was holding my hand. She looked worried, yet the kindliness in her face took away my fear. The first thought that came into my head was a scripture verse from the Old Testament book of Deuteronomy. God told Moses, "I will never leave you nor forsake you." Apparently, my heart had spontaneously started beating again on its own. When everyone was confident that my rhythm was stable, they withdrew and left me alone, safely connected to monitors that would signal any further trouble.

Moments later my mother called. I asked her to hang up the phone, call my husband, tell him that I had coded and ask him to come immediately. I must have scared her to death. I still feel terrible about upsetting her so, but I desperately needed to talk to Jim, to tell him I loved him.

Shortly after she hung up, my heart stopped beating for the second time. Just as has been documented by many other people who have had near-death experiences, I once again found myself traveling down a long, dark tunnel with a bright and comforting light at the end. It was neither frightening nor upsetting. In fact, it was very peaceful. There was no sound.

Again, when I woke up, Sister Katherine was holding my right hand and a physician's assistant was holding my left. I was hooked up to the defibrillator. Lots of people were crowded around my bed looking both concerned and relieved. Now I was frightened. The situation soon repeated itself one more time exactly like the first two: everyone left; I coded and woke up with Sister Katherine holding my hand. I will forever remember the reassurance of her presence, her attentiveness to me.

Months later, when Lauren came home for the holidays, she, Jim and I were talking about that day. Jim had arrived after the first code. Lauren and Brad arrived after the third code. They found their father alone, confused and crying in the waiting room. None of them yet had any idea what happened before they reached the hospital that day.

One of the doctors took time to come out of the unit and explain that I needed the ICD immediately implanted. There was a patient undergoing some type of procedure in a room on my own floor, and they would interrupt the procedure to make the room available for me. He said that my condition was extremely serious and if no one came out of the room within the first fifteen minutes, it would mean I was still alive. He was in a hurry, but his manner was professional and honest. Lauren, Brad and Jim were so traumatized by the seriousness of my condition that they couldn't even say a word to each other.

Hours later, the doctors encouraged my family to come into the Recovery Room to speak to me. The ICD was in and all had gone well. I don't remember anything else about that day. My mother and sister Mare – for Mary Ann – arrived later that afternoon to find my family in a state of shock. Lauren remembers feeling relieved by the presence of her aunt and her grandmother. She could share some of the burden. Spreading the pain out might make it hurt less.

Tuesday-Friday, August 28-31

The next several days were medically uneventful. I was grateful to be alive. I was thankful for the gifts and skills of the professionals who had saved my life. I praised God and the staff. I had the impression that I was cured, that in time I would surely get better and be fine again.

I received activity instructions for the long term. I could not drive a car for six months. I could never play golf again. (Neither directive made me very happy.) I was in a one-hundred percent pacer rhythm, which means that I had no beats of my own; my body was relying entirely on the implanted device.

A test of the ICD was scheduled for Friday. Essentially, the test is an induced code so that the physician has confidence that the device will function on demand as intended. I was frightened of the procedure. I'd already coded three times earlier in the week and wasn't looking forward to traveling down that tunnel again. I woke up crying, the procedure a success and the staff compassionate and kind. They gave me a few moments to pull myself together before wheeling me back through the halls on the stretcher, and into my bed. I remember their thoughtfulness to this day.

Sister Katherine accompanied me later that afternoon to the Pulmonary Function Lab. I was transported via wheelchair while attached to the portable monitor, so my heartbeat could be watched the whole time I was out of the unit. The ICD was regulating my heartbeat internally. The monitor allowed my heartbeat to be viewed externally real-time – a vital precaution.

While we were waiting, I asked Sister Katherine if we could review the strips of the codes, as she knew I was a nurse with a cardiac background. The monitor prints out a reading of the heart rhythm on a paper strip, like an ECG. The strips are placed in the patient's chart as a record of the event. My strips showed I had deteriorated from a complete heart block, where the atria and ventricles beat in a rhythm completely dissociated from each other, to flat line. There were several pages of six-second strips of flat line. If I hadn't been in the hospital, in a critical care step-down unit, attached to a cardiac monitor, within feet of a defibrillator and surrounded by trained professionals, I would not have survived. At that moment, I understood for the first time the gravity of my situation. The defibrillator was safely implanted and checked, and would be essential to my life.

Saturday-Monday, September 1-3, Labor Day Weekend

On Friday, my attending physicians had written discharge orders for me to go home that night. All of the physicians who had cared for me were apparently off for the holiday weekend. Most hospitals tend to send patients home on weekends – and especially holiday weekends – as staffing is light. The problem was that I did not feel well at all. And for the next several days I was to be visited regularly and examined by the partners of my admitting physicians.

Universally, *all* of these physicians encouraged me to go home, believing that in time I would feel better, and meanwhile I would truly be more comfortable there. But I said I didn't feel well and couldn't imagine going home feeling so poorly. Make no mistake about it; I'm no shrinking violet. My father has often teased me about being so tough. I have a high tolerance for pain, a trait that would serve me well over the months to follow.

A physician's assistant examined me on Saturday morning, and found that I was by then in heart failure and ordered intravenous Lasix, a diuretic. To my knowledge that was the first time I knew that I was in failure. Lasix causes one to diurese excess fluid from the vascular tree, which means a million trips to the bathroom. Later that day, I was transferred to a medical-surgical telemetry unit.

I was placed on another type of portable heart monitor, which allowed the nurses to view my heartbeat out at their workstation. My roommate was a blind, elderly woman who did not speak. The nurses kept the television on twenty-four hours a day to keep her company. I was exhausted. I am a noise- and light-sensitive person. I could not sleep in a room with a television running twenty-four hours a day. I asked the nurses to turn it off but they perhaps understandably refused, as they were thinking what would be best for the elderly patient. I understood, but it was not the best situation for me. Without adequate sleep I continued to go downhill.

Each day over that long weekend my attending physician, a kind and thoughtful man, would come into the room in the morning, examine me with care and ask if I was ready to go home. The heart failure issue seemed to have resolved! Despite how unrestful the room was, however, I did not feel well and I was afraid to go home. Gently he explained that given all I had gone through the previous week, it was not unexpected that I would feel this way. Further, he cautioned, it might take time for me to feel better. Each day, when I considered how I felt, I thought it best to stay a little longer.

Finally, on the third day, even though I didn't feel appreciably better, I decided to go home. At least, I thought, I would get more rest in my own bed. And sincerely, the medical staff believed it was safe for me to be discharged.

Jim and Brad picked me up and home I went. I remember telephoning the doctor on call at bedtime to tell him I just did not feel right; nothing I could pinpoint, just a vague sense of doom. The physician on call was another member of the practice whom I did not know. He said firmly "go to the Emergency Room," and hung up. It was the correct advice, but delivered without a sense of caring. I felt alone and absolutely defeated.

Months later, stabilized and reflective, I would write a letter to my original, extremely competent admitting physician at the hospital. I confessed that in the drama of all the events that unfolded so quickly throughout my hospitalization, neither my family nor I remember any conversation about my prognosis long term. I asked what he had determined my diagnosis to be and what he had expected my recovery to be. I asked if he had had any inkling that my case would turn out to be so unusual.

My doctor explained that my disease was so extremely rare he could not have predicted the later diagnosis, nor the outcome. He went on to say it wasn't likely the hospital would ever see the disease again, but that they knew more now because of what happened to me. In fact, they treated the statistically most probable disease, viral myocarditis, itself a rare and often difficult to recognize disease with only 4,000 cases in the United States per year. (I had to admit that their rationale was absolutely on target. The fact that anyone, anywhere would recognize my disease, giant cell myocarditis, would be just one of many miracles to come.) According to standard medical practice, most patients with my symptoms do indeed recover completely from viral myocarditis without any residual dysfunction. With rest, time, medication and the supportive device, I should have recovered.

Tuesday, September 4

The next morning was Tuesday, the day after Labor Day. We quickly realized I wasn't well enough to be left alone and therefore Jim could not go back to work. My sister Mare and her two dogs arrived later that afternoon with the intention of staying with me for the remainder of the week. It was not to be so.

Around dinnertime, I was on the phone with Lauren when I suddenly realized I felt exceedingly unwell. I told her I had to go. I asked Mare and Jim to call 911. I couldn't feel any radial pulses.

The policeman arrived first, followed shortly by the local volunteer rescue squad. Our dog Ruffie and my sister's two dogs formed a protective ring around me as they sensed that the uniformed workers were there to take me away. Ruffie grabbed the pants-leg of the policeman and yanked. Given that Ruffie weighs only about twenty pounds, the scene was in retrospect quite comical. My sister's Jack Russell terrier sat on my chest growling at the rescue workers. Her yellow lab Harley wagged her tail for our guests, but the hair on her neck was standing straight up. The whole scene was "organized chaos." The dogs did give way at last.

The squad members made several attempts to take my blood pressure but were unsuccessful, so they quickly completed their paperwork, assuming that as often happens the blood pressure cuffs were malfunctioning. They loaded me into the ambulance and we raced off to the Huntington Hospital Emergency Room.

I remember things happening quickly once I got to the ER. I had the full attention of the nursing and medical staff. I had no discernible blood pressure. Jim reached over to rub my leg and I shouted, "Don't touch me!" I was burning up. I was thrashing in the bed as if I'd been injected with Speed.

The staff couldn't get intravenous lines in to my veins or draw blood. I knew I was on the brink of death. From the looks on the faces of my family and the medical staff I knew my situation was grave. I made them cut off my nightgown because I was too sick to struggle with removing it over my head. I vomited and was incontinent of feces and urine. For the first and only time in my life, I prayed that God would take me. I was wild with fear, with adrenaline coursing through my veins – as my body fought to save itself.

My family physician was not on call that evening. His covering physician Dr.

Charles Mascioli was brought in by the ER staff to manage my case. Dr. Mascioli turned out to be an angel in disguise. He never left my side for the remainder of the night. I remember the look of concern and fear on his face. He called in a cardiologist, another physician who was not mine, to consult on my case. He too never left my side. He too looked frightened.

Though I don't remember much else about the next several hours, Jim tells me they told him gently and straightforwardly that it was likely I would not live – but if through some miracle I did, my only chance for survival was a heart transplant. Months later, in a conversation with my doctor from St. Francis, I learned that they had called him swiftly to seek advice, as St. Francis's specialty is interventional cardiology, which includes surgery for coronary vessel disease. A diagnosis of cardiomyopathy – deterioration of the heart muscle – might require the heart transplant. They were told that there was nothing further St. Francis could do for me and that in fact, a stop at St. Francis for a cardiac biopsy would be dangerous to me. It was recommended that I be transported directly to Manhattan's NewYork-Presbyterian Hospital/Columbia (NYPH/C) for a possible heart transplant.

Huntington Hospital needed to stabilize my blood pressure, however, before I could be transported. Jim said they worked assiduously for hours trying different medications and combinations of medications to stabilize the pressure, which by now had dropped to a near-lethal 60 over 20 mmHg. And then, as if by magic, I developed a safer blood pressure of 80mmHg over something. With Dr. Mascioli and the cardiologist at my side, I would soon be transported to the CCU to await EMT transportation to NewYork-Presbyterian.

One of Huntington's CCU nurses, who I remember promised to pray for me, had me sign a Living Will, which designated my husband and my sister as having the authority to make decisions about my care if I was incompetent to do so. She talked to me with honesty and respect. She cared for me like a piece of priceless fine china. She held my hand, stroking it as she softly spoke. She stayed by my side. She was not afraid to face death with me. I will never forget her.

My family physician, the one for whom Dr. Mascioli had been on call, came to the unit and stood quietly at the door of my room. His sadness at their being unable to provide the help I needed left a chasm as wide as the Grand Canyon. The decision was made to transfer me for more specialized care.

Huntington's cardiologist promptly called the hospital operator at NYPH/C in the middle of the night and was given the home phone number of one of the hospital's famous heart transplant physicians. He asked Dr. Oz if they could take me on as a patient and Dr. Oz simply said, "Bring her in."

❦

"One of Huntington's CCU nurses, who I remember promised to pray for me, had me sign a Living Will, which designated my husband and my sister as having the authority to make decisions about my care if I was incompetent to do so. She talked to me with honesty and respect. She cared for me like a piece of priceless fine china. She held my hand, stroking it as she softly spoke. She stayed by my side. She was not afraid to face death with me. I will never forget her. . . ."

"Huntington's cardiologist promptly called the hospital operator at NYPH/C in the middle of the night and was given the home phone number of one of the hospital's famous heart transplant physicians. He asked Dr. Oz if they could take me on as a patient and Dr. Oz simply said, 'Bring her in.'"

———————————————

"God is our refuge and strength,
a very present help in trouble." – Psalm 46:1

———— ❤ ————

3 SURRENDERING MY HEART

Wednesday, September 5, 2001

I went by ambulance to NewYork-Presbyterian Hospital/Columbia and was admitted directly to the Critical Coronary Care Unit, an eighteen-bed unit on the fifth floor of the NYPH/C Milstein Building. This unit was to become my home for the next four weeks, and the staff would become my family.

As I was being moved from the stretcher to my bed, Jim was introduced to Dr. Mario Deng, one of the transplant physicians, who said to my husband, "I certainly hope your wife does not have anything so esoteric as giant cell myocarditis." Jim sensed immediately that he regretted saying that out loud – not that we had any idea what the implications were of such a diagnosis, just that it was not good.

A cardiac biopsy, performed the next day, proved Dr. Deng's fear well founded. As soon as the diagnosis was made, the physicians on the NYPH/C Heart Failure Team started calling medical institutions around the country to find out how they had treated this disease, and with what success.

Giant cell myocarditis is a rare and most often fatal autoimmune disease that affects young and otherwise healthy individuals. Its cause is not usually known, but two factors sometimes play an important role in accurately diagnosing the disease. It requires that an individual have a genetic predisposition to autoimmune dysfunction, as well as some sort of environmental trigger. Asthma is itself an autoimmune disease. Looking back, I realize I must have inherited this genetic predisposition to autoimmune dysfunction from my father, who has long had a pacemaker for cardiomyopathy. I believe his heart was damaged each time he coded during surgery as a result of his own hypersensitivity reactions to anesthesia.

In giant cell myocarditis, the literature documents that patients have reported a variety of environmental triggers – ranging from hypersensitivity reactions to immunizations or medications, the presence of foreign bodies, pregnancy, bacterial and viral infections and a disparate set of diseases. At the time of my diagnosis at NewYork-Presbyterian Hospital/Columbia, there had as noted been only two hundred cases reported worldwide since the 1905 report. NYPH/C had seen two cases in the past eleven years. Dr. Deng had seen one case when he was practicing in Germany years prior to emigrating to the United States. The patient died prior to transplantation, despite being supported by a left ventricular assist device.

I have since learned plenty about this fearsome diagnosis – that giant cell myocarditis is essentially a pathological diagnosis with a rapidly deteriorating clinical course.

> *"Clinically, patients experience malignant tachyarrhythmias [interpreted to mean fast and irregular], profound heart failure and rapid demise."*
>
> – "Giant Cell Myocarditis as a Manifestation of Drug Hypersensitivity," Paul R. Daniels, M.D., et al

> *"The cause of this rare disease is not known. The median time from symptom onset to presentation is 3 weeks. The median age is 42 years of age. Men and women are affected equally, and cases have been described in many ethnic groups. . . . Without*

transplantation, prognosis is poor. The time to death or heart transplantation is five months. Most patients die before ever having their names placed on a transplant list. The diagnosis is often made on autopsy. I suspect that many patients have died and continue to die of this disease because they were never accurately diagnosed due to a lack of availability of cardiac biopsy or the lack of awareness in the medical community of this disease. Post transplant survival is approximately 71% at 5 years despite a 25% rate of recurrence in the new heart."

– Dr. Leslie T. Cooper, Jr.

"*Pathologically speaking, the diagnosis is made by documenting the presence of multinucleated giant cells amidst a diffuse and multifocal inflammatory infiltrate.*"

– "Giant Cell Myocarditis: Diagnosis and Treatment,"
Dr. Leslie T. Cooper, Jr.

In other words, the muscle tissue of the heart is inflamed and the tissue under microscope is populated with these otherwise nonexistent giant cells. It's like having an infection in or on any other part of your body: the tissue swells and becomes red hot. The doctors said my heart was huge. Because my heart was inflamed and huge, it could not perform its function of providing oxygenated blood to my body, therefore I was in heart failure. I did not have a viable blood pressure even with several potent intravenous heart-strengthening and anti-hypotensive drugs and fluid was backing up out of the vascular tree and into my lungs. Unmistakably, I was in critical condition.

In the Critical Coronary Care Unit at NYPH/C, I was hooked up to every conceivable form of monitoring device. As I lay in bed I was the audience for a cacophony of bells, whistles, alarms and pneumonic devices. I had arterial lines in my wrist, the pacemaker/defibrillator device in my chest wall, intravenous lines in my arms, PIC lines (type of IV) into my arm, central venous pressure lines in my neck, a cardiac monitor on my chest, oxygen in my nose and a Foley catheter in my bladder. I had x-rays, blood draws, cardiac biopsies, ECG's, echocardiograms and MUGA scans (where they test heart function by injecting a radioactive solution into a patient's veins and then take pictures of the heart) – and some of those tests were repeated daily. I look back on all this with wonder: so much danger, so fast, from such a simple wish – to go to Malawi to help the less fortunate.

So there I was, all hooked up in CCU. As a nurse I knew perfectly well how to read the monitors. I knew what the blood pressure values meant. I knew my arterial blood was not supposed to be brown. I knew my life was hanging in the balance. I knew the doctors were doing everything they could. I knew that whether I lived or died my life was in God's hands.

Every time I fell asleep, I was surprised to wake up. Most importantly, and I remember so clearly this absolute realization, I knew that God was with me. When I closed my eyes, I saw a textured, rust-colored curtain with a bright light behind it. I had the sense that God was behind that curtain, His light so intense, His power so immense that it could not be viewed directly, but His presence was with me. When I focused on His presence, I was truly not afraid.

Every time I viewed my son's face, his pain so palpable, I was overcome with grief. When he kissed me goodnight every night before he went home or to the waiting room to sleep in a chair, I did not know if I would see him again. My husband was stunned. My daughter was sunshine and smiles, doing her best to put on a good face for me, trying hard not to let me see her pain, trying hard to keep the family from falling apart. Months later, and only when her job was done, she would fall apart herself.

My sister and my brother came every day too. We are a very close family, but this was the biggest challenge any of us had ever faced. My mother brought me food. It is no secret that hospital cuisine leaves something to be desired, so my mother did what she does best: she brought me good, healthy things to eat. I did not have an appetite and I was losing weight but she brought me food. My dad couldn't come at all because he was still in the rehabilitation hospital receiving therapy for his knee replacement. What a time, what a surprise, this illness. And yet what immeasurable love it brought forth.

"Every time I fell asleep, I was surprised to wake up. Most importantly, and I remember so clearly this absolute realization, I knew that God was with me. When I closed my eyes, I saw a textured, rust-colored curtain with a bright light behind it. I had the sense that God was behind that curtain, His light so intense, His power so immense that it could not be viewed directly, but His presence was with me. When I focused on His presence, I was truly not afraid. . . ."

*"In the Critical Coronary Care Unit at NYPH/C, I was hooked
up to every conceivable form of monitoring device. As I lay in bed I was the
audience for a cacophony of bells, whistles, alarms and pneumonic
devices. I had arterial lines in my wrist, the pacemaker/defibrillator device in
my chest wall, intravenous lines in my arms, PIC lines (type of IV)
into my arm, central venous pressure lines in my neck, a cardiac monitor on
my chest, oxygen in my nose and a Foley catheter in my bladder. I
had x-rays, blood draws, cardiac biopsies, ECG's, echocardiograms and
MUGA scans (where they test heart function by injecting a
radioactive solution into a patient's veins and then take pictures of the heart)
– and some of those tests were repeated daily. I look back on
all this with wonder: so much danger, so fast, from such a simple wish
– to go to Malawi to help the less fortunate. . . ."*

"For where your treasure is,
there your heart will be also." – Matthew 6:21

—— 💜 ——

4 AUGUST-SEPTEMBER 2001 . . . SEASON OF CHANGE: A DAUGHTER'S PERSPECTIVE

August-September, 2001

I write about this time one year later, remembering those first weeks of my mother's frightening challenge. The fall has always been a time of major change for me. I grew up on the East Coast in a small town in New Jersey. Despite its unfavorable reputation in most parts of the country, New Jersey was an incredible place to grow up. We had the ocean in the summer, the mountains in the winter, and New York City about forty minutes away. Probably my favorite part of childhood, and consequently what I miss most now that I live in California, is the changing of the four seasons. The activities you do, the foods you eat, the places you visit all move through a cyclical set of changes with nature. Oddly, summer tended to be my least favorite time of year, followed by my favorite, fall. Summer always seemed to carry the baggage from the year before and an expectation of the most fun. By August I could not wait for change.

The funny thing about change is that it is essential for growth. It is futile for us to fight change, and it always brings a new understanding, which is definitely a positive thing. In my own experience, however, there are always incredibly hard times that lead up to the climax; if there is a harder way to learn new lessons I always seem to find it. But sometimes it finds me.

It was a typical day at work, that mid-August afternoon when Mom's first call came. I was a field sales person in the electronics industry in Silicon Valley. My business had just been getting up and running when the bottom fell out of the economy. I got pretty sick of meeting after meeting with everyone asking "When is this going to end?" but otherwise I was still really enjoying myself. I had earned a good reputation with both the people I worked with in my company, and my counterparts in other companies. Everyone told me I just needed to weather the economic storm and I could write my own ticket. In the meantime, I was happy with my salary and with my schedule. Life was flying by.

But things were changing as summer began to end. I was starting to question what I was still doing in Santa Cruz after graduating from the University more than two years earlier. I was paying too much in rent and I was partying too hard. I felt pulled along by the tides. I couldn't separate myself from my own situation enough to question what path I was on.

I have always been very close to my mom and dad and brother. We have a pretty idyllic relationship. Although my parents live on Long Island and my brother in New Jersey we talk all the time and take numerous trips each year to be together. That's why it was no surprise when I got a call in the early afternoon that Friday in August from my mom. In fact, it wasn't even a total shock that my mom was calling from the Huntington Hospital emergency room. She had developed asthma a couple of years before and due to her extreme sensitivity to all kinds of medication, she has had to go to the hospital on several occasions to monitor her reactions and adjust her medication.

Mom was explaining that she had been pretty tired from being with my grandfather all week, after his second knee replacement in a couple of years. My mom was always the caretaker to everyone, especially her family. In many long conversations throughout the years we always talked about the way she gives so much of herself that she sometimes leaves nothing for herself. Being my mom's cheerleader, I always try to encourage her to do more for herself. But, being her daughter and knowing how wonderful her gifts are, I was guilty of accepting her offerings as well.

My mom was born as a giving person and she's always found religion an affirmation of her generosity. That day when she called, she had no idea she was about to begin one situation in life where she had nothing to give and needed all the prayer and support she could get.

On the phone, my mom spoke of an irregular heartbeat and an uncomfortable feeling in her chest. I was instantly reminded of all of the rapid heartbeats she had felt with reactions to her asthma medication. I asked if she needed me to come out and be with her but she refused, saying she would be fine. I went on with my weekend plans and figured that as usual she would discover an overdose of medication or an undiagnosed reaction to medication.

Then Saturday morning I received another call. Mom said that doctors at St. Francis Hospital had recorded something irregular in her heart rhythm and they were going to do a test on Sunday where they would try to replicate the heart rhythms through drugs. She asked that I fly out for the procedure.

I felt scared and very strange about considering the potential frailty of my mom's health. I remembered hearing about a friend's father suffering a heart attack, and she sobbed all night despite the comfort of many who cared. I felt instantly removed and somehow different from my own friends, but nowhere in need of a shoulder to cry on. The trip to me seemed more of an inconvenience to my job and my social life, yet a family obligation that I was more than happy to meet.

Incredibly, looking back, Saturday morning turned into Saturday afternoon and I found myself almost resenting this family obligation to leave my life in Santa Cruz. Then I got a call from Dad telling me to either get on a plane within the next two hours or not see Mom until after her procedure on Sunday.

Still not realizing the magnitude of the situation, I was leaning toward the later flight. Mom was always very clear at letting me know what I should do and what not, but with Dad things weren't always so clear. Maybe my first inkling of the seriousness of the situation was the fact that Dad insisted I take the earlier flight to see Mom on Saturday night before the procedure. It was supposed to be one where the physicians induce an unusual reaction in the heart. Mom was nervous because she didn't like the thought of them artificially messing around with her heart rate. I did take the earlier flight, for which I will always be grateful.

My dad picked me up at the airport. I admire my dad almost more than anyone. He is so smart, handsome, athletic, professional and classy, but still cool. We have a deep mutual respect for one another but don't talk the way my mom and I do. He's the type of guy you always want close in an emergency. He is very competent, and even as his family we knew how well he did managing crises in his business life. He seemed edgy and very matter of fact as we drove from JFK airport out to the hospital on Long Island.

Seeing Mom instantly made me feel better. Her face always lit up when she saw me, and although she was in a hospital gown in bed, she looked good. We chatted for awhile and she expressed her concern for the following day, but also shared the reassuring words that the doctors had given her. This was just a test and should give them the information they needed to accurately diagnose her condition. In retrospect, the test that had us all so worried seems insignificant, in light of all that would follow.

The test showed irregularities in her heart function. For a forty-nine-year-old woman in excellent physical condition, who never smoked and rarely drank anything at all, her heart problems were due not to clogged arteries but to electrical problems. So the doctors felt that my mom needed a special pacemaker to help keep her electrical impulses even and her heart function normal.

She was nervous about the operation and the need for the device – which some nurses told her might limit her ability to drive, but overall relieved to learn that the situation was treatable. She was scheduled for surgery the next morning and expected to go home within a few days for the Labor Day holiday weekend. I called work and told them I'd be another two days and changed my plane tickets.

The next morning my father headed into the hospital early to spend time with Mom before her surgery. My brother Brad and I did some grocery shopping for Dad so he'd have food in the house during the week and when Mom came home that weekend. We arrived at the hospital about an hour and a half after my father to a sight that I will never forget. It was an image that set the tone for how serious a situation my mother was really in.

My father was at the end of the hall, just around the corner from where I knew my mom's room was, crying, with a nun consoling him. Having never seen my father cry before, I knew something serious was going down. Dad told my brother and me that he had been holding Mom's hand and comforting her when her eyes rolled back in her head and her heart monitor showed she was flat-lining. He said that the system hooked up to her heart let out loud alarms and doctors and nurses came running out of nowhere and pushed him aside. This time, they had to use the defibrillator to shock her body back to life. After her pulse regained some strength and they had called her physicians, my dad was allowed back into the room. He said she was really scared but didn't remember much about what had happened. They talked for a minute or two and he consoled her and then she flat-lined again. Immediately a team of nurses surrounded her bed and my dad was escorted to the hall, which is where we found him.

The three of us and the nun – who did her best to tell us everything would be all right even though we all knew that things were far from it – headed into the waiting room just down the hall from Mom to wait for the doctor. The doctor told us that although this morning's episodes were serious, they only further confirmed his opinion that the ICD was what she needed.

The problem, however, was getting the device in before she coded again. First they had to get her into an operating room as quickly as possible. We were told that there was only one operating room on her floor, and they were moving a patient out to open it up for her. We were told that we had only fifteen minutes to worry about her. Within that time they would have the device in, and she would be safe.

The three of us sat in a small waiting room in the cardiology unit of St. Francis Hospital with the nun – Sister Katherine as we would learn. We stared at the clock. You can't read or watch TV at a time like that. All I wanted to do was to call a friend. I knew he was at work and his cell phone never connected when he was at his job site. I didn't care that I probably wouldn't get through; I had to try. The only pay phone on the floor was being used. I stood a respectful distance away and waited for the gentleman to finish. As time passed and my desperation mounted I couldn't do anything but stand in the middle of all of the people passing by, and cry. The man saw me and never got off the phone.

Noticing, Sister Katherine asked if I wanted to use her phone. On the first try, I got through to my friend and told him the whole story through my tears. I needed to tell him, to feel his friendship, to lessen the pain a little by sharing it with someone else. I told him I'd call him when I heard anything else and headed back into the waiting room. His words were a great comfort to me.

After the forty-five minutes we all assumed the operation was a success, and soon the doctors told us she was in recovery and everything had gone smoothly. They let us see her fairly quickly. I remember how weak and fragile she looked in the hospital bed. She was barely awake, and maybe it was her groggy appearance or the rush of a day of intense emotions, but I felt dark corners close in on my vision. My face felt hot and cold at the same time and everything seemed to slow down. I had to go into the hallway with my brother to keep from passing out.

The next day Mom seemed a bit better and the doctors were still optimistic that she would be sent home that weekend. I kept my plans to head home the next day to get back to work, and maybe to try to make some sense of all that had happened. I was both sad and relieved to be leaving; it was a feeling I would have many times that fall and I would feel guilty every time.

I worked the day after I returned to California and was looking forward to the holiday weekend myself. I can remember stopping by another friend's house the next night, and telling him the story of what had happened to my mom in the previous days. He was not a particularly close friend, but I found myself quite calmly telling him the whole story. I must not even have looked up at him until I was finished and was surprised to see him crying. It would be the first of many times I'd be able to realize the pain I was feeling only by the expressions on others' faces, as I shared my experiences. I think that when shocking things happen to people it takes some time for their emotions to catch up. Either that, or someplace inside of yourself you realize that you can't deal with what you feel, you can only go through the motions of life.

My mom was released from the hospital sometime that holiday weekend and I remember being surprised that she wasn't more excited about it. She told me in phone conversations from her hospital bed that she was scared that if something happened to her while she was home, no one would be there to save her. I felt she was probably just shaken up from her experiences, but I also knew better than to pass off my mom's intuition as just fear. At this point, though, we were all so freaked out by the whole intense and sudden crisis, that maybe we all just wanted to believe it was over.

I was on the phone with Mom the day after she went home. My Aunt Mare had come out to take care of her and they were having dinner with my dad. Mom sounded good but distracted. Very abruptly she told me she needed to get off the phone. I asked why, and was concerned because of how unlike her it was not to end every conversation with about twenty "I love you's." She just said she needed to go and hung up.

I got a call from Dad two hours later. He was very distressed. Mom had begun having chest pain while she was on the phone with me and asked him to call 911. The paramedics rushed her to the local emergency room where doctors spent hours trying to keep her alive with various combinations of medicines. Her blood pressure dropped very low. My mom's body sensed it was in a crisis situation and began producing adrenaline to fight to stay alive. My dad said she was writhing from the discomfort and intense heat.

What a frightening call that was. We agreed to talk again as soon as possible. After Mom had stabilized, the emergency room doctor on staff that night pulled my father aside. He asked him if he knew how sick my mom really was and if anyone had talked to him about the possibility of her needing a heart transplant. He said that using everything he knew he was barely able to keep her alive, and that he had to get her out of his hospital to a place better able to help her. He had called NewYork-Presbyterian Hospital/Columbia in Manhattan and was having her sent there tomorrow by ambulance. A team of physicians would review her entire medical history prior to her arriving, and work on a possible diagnosis.

I stood there in shock and frustration and fear, trying to comprehend the magnitude of all this. Next my father told me something that to this day he does not remember saying, but I can still hear it in my ears and I know why this dear man needed to say it. He said that I needed to come to terms with the fact that Mom might not make it through this. He said I would need to be strong, because he was doing all he could to be there for her and he would not be able to be a shoulder for me to cry on. This message was a reflection of just how serious a situation my mom was in. It was not something that my dad could protect me from. I kept it together and did stay strong while we were on the phone. Later, I cried myself to sleep.

I caught a plane back to JKF the following day. It was a long transcontinental flight and I had to catch a cab at the airport because my brother Brad and my father were already at the hospital with Mom. I hit a ton of traffic and the cab driver got lost on the way. By the time I reached the hospital uptown in Manhattan, I had been traveling for almost twelve hours.

I walked into my mom's room and she looked at me and, without expression, looked away. At that moment I knew how sick she really was. My mom is one of those women who loves her children with every cell in her body. She says that my brother and I are her two greatest accomplishments and she has spent a lifetime being the most generous, loving, supportive, and encouraging mother I have ever known. I'm not sure which hurt more: to know that Mom was not thinking of her love for me, or to know she was in so much discomfort that she wasn't even herself. When I bring this day up to her now, she doesn't remember reacting this way.

As my mom has since written in her own story, the team of physicians diagnosed her with a very rare autoimmune disease, giant cell myocarditis. They believe the disease was triggered by vaccinations received in preparation for her trip to Africa to raise money for children with AIDS. The vaccines, combined with her sensitivity to medications and her overactive immune system, gave her a disease that the hospital had seen only twice in its history.

Life presents us with so many messages if only we are listening. This is one that continues to both baffle and reveal itself to my family and me in so many ways. How could a very religious woman – who has devoted her life to her faith and her family and has taken care of her own health and the health of others – contract a highly fatal, extremely rare disease triggered by her desire to help under-privileged children dying in a health epidemic? In the months that followed I per-sonally would struggle with my own understanding of life and my faith, trying to make sense of this time.

My mother's fiftieth birthday fell on Monday, September 10, 2001. I had spent a rough weekend with her and yet was scheduled to fly back to resume my own life the day after her birthday. Mom's health was precarious, and the hardest thing was to watch her own understanding of the situation. Having been an inten-sive care unit nurse for years, she understood the results of her tests and monitors better than the rest of us.

We all spent long ten-hour days in her room telling funny family stories and leaving the room only for a bite to eat in the cafeteria, or to give other relatives a chance to visit. I would go home to Long Island with my father at night to feed the dog and cat, eat something, answer the multitude of messages from friends and family inquiring about Mom.

My mother was so sick that she asked that only her immediate family visit her in the hospital. Flowers were not permitted in her wing of the hospital because of the bacteria and germs they could carry to patients. Many friends felt helpless about how they could offer support. Dad was often so spent by the end of the day that he couldn't call everyone back. We would usually call one or two people and ask them to send cards for us to bring to Mom, and to pass the message along to others.

This weekend, Mom felt so sick that she asked that I leave first thing Monday morning and not stay later for her birthday. My aunt and grandmother made her special food that day, but she was so sick from her caustic cocktail of medications that she couldn't eat.

I took an early flight around 8 a.m. on September 10 and arrived in time to work a half-day at my office. In a sales position, your consistency and availability for customers is crucial to your success. Missing so much time and being so distracted when I was there was affecting my accounts; I was doing my best to get in front of customers as much as possible. Sometimes when people asked about my mom I would answer very matter-of-factly about her most recent reports and status, but other times I would simply break down and cry. There was a growing mound of pain and emotion inside of me that I knew I had no time to release. I rarely cried during these weeks; I believe I was too sad even to cry.

I was planning on going into work a little late on Tuesday, the 11th, and was surprised to get a phone call from a girlfriend at work telling me that a plane had crashed into one of the towers of the World Trade Center in New York. She told me the phone lines were all busy and I probably wouldn't be able to reach my family. I ran to the TV and sat on the floor about three feet from the screen, trying to comprehend the scene I was watching. I saw the second plane crash into the second tower, and I watched as both towers fell soon after.

The TV news was reporting that any non-critical patients would be moved from New York area hospitals to make room for the expected casualties from the towers. My mom later told me that although she was barely aware of what was going on, she knew she was one of the only patients on her floor not considered eligible for transfer. In time I got calls from my family and learned everyone was safe. My mom had been so sick the night before that my father and my brother spent the night in the hospital and they were there with her, which was wonderful. The thought of her being all alone without family was unbearable.

I went to work later that day and found it hard to look up from the floor. I was having such a hard time comprehending the intense tragedy that had struck the nation and my family simultaneously. One thought kept coming back to me – all of those lost in the Twin Towers didn't even stand a chance of survival. So many never made it to hospitals or even ambulances. Most of the victims had gone to work that morning as healthy, normal people while my Mom lay dying in a hospital bed. So many families had been happy and healthy over the preceding weeks, while mine was sick and scared. But at the end of the day they were dead and my mom was still fighting for her life.

– Lauren A. Moose
August-September 2002

♥

"I can remember stopping by another friend's house the next night,
and telling him the story of what had happened to my mom in the previous
days. He was not a particularly close friend, but I found myself
quite calmly telling him the whole story. I must not even have looked up at
him until I was finished and was surprised to see him crying. It would
be the first of many times I'd be able to realize the pain I was feeling only by
the expressions on others' faces, as I shared my experiences. . . ."

"My flesh and my heart fail; but God is the strength of my heart and my portion forever." – Psalm 73:26

5 THE FAILING HEART

Sometime in early September, 2001

I don't remember each day as clearly as I do the events leading up to this point. I was still desperately ill and perhaps thankfully do not remember every detail. The ICD was in but my heart still was failing. Periodically the NewYork-Presbyterian physicians would order tests to evaluate the function of my heart. The results showed continuing decline.

There was a routine of sorts to the next five weeks of my hospitalization. The junior medical staff performed their pre-rounds physical assessment of me at 5 a.m. The phlebotomist drew blood every morning at 6 a.m. Breakfast trays were delivered at 8:30. Then lunch at noon, dinner at 5. ECG's and chest x-rays were also performed before noon. The nurses handed out oral and intravenous medications at intervals throughout the day. Physicians from every specialty and every academic level came and went from my room, as if by revolving door, each performing a particular task that it was hoped would contribute to my health.

I remember that there were so many staffmembers who touched me in special ways. Each took care to connect with me on a personal level, a wonderful combination of skill and caring. I viewed each of them as a gift from God sent to give me strength and encouragement. They were wonderful people – they cared so much, they made a point of getting to know me. They lingered. They told me about themselves (they already knew everything about me!). I mattered to them. Without them, I couldn't have made it through.

My mother, sister Mare and cousin Jan would visit at noon almost every day. Jim would go to work most mornings and leave at noon to come to my bedside until he wasn't allowed to stay. My son Brad came every evening after work, stayed at the hospital, slept in the waiting room or a motel and drove out of the City in the morning. He showered at work in the gym and then put in a full day, only to repeat the process every day for almost two months.

My wonderful brother Sam, who is a very busy veterinarian in a solo practice, would visit every evening while his wife and brand new baby spent hours in the waiting room alone. Sam would bring fresh tomatoes from his garden for all of the nurses on all of the shifts, which they adored. When the seasons progressed into fall, he brought baskets of apples for the staff as well. He is a very big, very handsome, very warm and outgoing guy. As with Mare and Jan, a light of healing emanated from him. I drew strength from his physical presence and his love. His children Matt and Rob (for Robin Sue), my nephew and niece, came often and stayed as long as they could. They were *with* me, despite how terribly painful my illness was for them. At this point, commercial planes were either not allowed to fly or reserved for only emergencies. Lauren was unable to visit for a number of weeks, and with no phone allowed in CCU, our communication was limited to messages sent through family members.

I met a coterie of medical professionals, doctors and nurses, as well as non-professionals of every level and representing different departments of the hospital. Each one visited my bedside, each assigned a task to perform. I tried to get to know them personally. Millie delivered the breakfast trays. Martina performed the ECG's. Andy, a medical student, inserted the intravenous lines. Dr. Yang, the chief resident, inserted the CVP and arterial lines. Susan, Remy and Jessie and many others whose names I cannot remember now were a few of the exceedingly skilled nurses who staff the CCU unit. I surrendered myself to their care and was confident that everything possible was being done to make me well. My life was hanging in the balance. It was important to me to connect with them as people. The personal connection, their caring for me as a human being, I believe, made all the difference in the world.

Dr. Rachel Remen, a physician herself, says in her book *My Grandfather's Blessings*, "Perhaps we can only truly serve those we are willing to touch, not only with our hands but with our hearts and even our souls. Professionalism has embedded in service a sense of difference, a certain distance. But on the deepest level, service is an experience of belonging, an experience of connection to others and to the world around us. It is this connection that gives us the power to bless the life in others. Without it, the life in them would not respond to us."

I decided I was going to be the best patient that this NYPH/C unit had ever had. I would not complain. I would not give in to pain. I would be compliant, generous, kind and supportive. I wanted to make the staff's care for me as easy as it could be. Being a nurse, I knew how much it hurts medical professionals to see people suffer. I prayed for the medical staff that struggled to insert all these lines. Because I was in heart failure, I had no peripheral pulses so they could not locate vessels to insert lines into. Several groups of physicians had been working on various parts of my body at different times, trying unsuccessfully to insert an arterial line, to monitor my blood oxygen level. They tried repeatedly and apologized profusely for hurting me. I prayed for them, that they would be successful, so they wouldn't feel so badly about hurting me.

Among many who cared for me so compassionately, I especially remember the young medical student Andy. He asked me to call him by his first name. He was extremely bright, and inexperienced yet so incredibly compassionate that he spoke to my heart. Andy had a challenge in finding my essentially vanished artery. He sought the advice of a more experienced colleague, who suggested an alternative technique that would be more painful for me, but had a greater chance of success. Andy explained everything to me in detail, mindful of the pain he would be causing me, and asked if I could withstand what he had to do. I said yes, and gently and carefully he did what was needed. I believe he soon rotated off cardiology service and I never saw him again. But I will remember him always. He will be a great doctor someday.

One of my heart failure physicians and his senior resident performed their assessment of my status daily. I knew by the look on their faces that they were concerned. I was touched by their humanity. Over the weeks that followed, they were not able to hide their sadness in my lack of progress. I could see it in their eyes. Yet throughout this time, I remember, they so clearly cared for me that I felt at peace. I surrendered to their skill, knowing that my life was in their caring and capable hands.

Monday, September 10

For the entire year leading up to this day, my mother had asked me what I wanted to do to celebrate my fiftieth birthday, a milestone to be sure. The birthday was not all that important to me, but our thirtieth wedding anniversary in June of the following year was. We are a family that celebrates all these important events. Some families do and some don't, but we do.

Certainly, I never expected to be "celebrating" my birthday in the hospital, critically ill. My sister brought a collage of pictures to post on the wall at the foot of my bed. One picture was of my dog Ruffie, and the rest were of my family.

Today was to be a first of a different sort as well. This day was my first treatment with chemotherapy. After calling all the major medical centers in the country Dr. Deng, who would become my post-transplant cardiologist, had decided to offer me participation in a clinical trial being conducted out of the Mayo Clinic in Rochester, Minnesota, by lead investigator Dr. Leslie Cooper. Dr. Cooper had been studying and writing about giant cell myocarditis for many years since his student days at Stanford University. He is now a world-renowned researcher and lecturer and is the country's leading expert on giant cell. I have earlier included excerpts from his research articles.

Dr. Deng had been in conversation with Dr. Cooper about my case. Together they decided I was not a candidate for inclusion in the study after all, because one of the drugs in the treatment protocol might be harmful to me, so a modified treatment plan was devised using both oral and intravenous therapies.

I was frightened to receive chemotherapy. My mother had barely survived her treatment for non-Hodgkin's lymphoma; it had been painful to watch her suffer and waste away. Throughout my own illness, I had tried so hard to let my husband be free from living at my bedside to perform his new job. Jim had a brand new company to run. He came almost every day to be at my bedside after he had put in some time in the office. Because I approached this new treatment with such trepidation, however, I asked him to stay overnight with me. The nurses let Jim and Brad alternate sleeping in the chair at the bedside, or sleeping on the floor in the waiting room with the other families who had desperately ill loved ones in the unit.

My cousin Jan had given me a Unity Church tape on healing to play while the medicine was being infused. The voice on the tape encouraged me to visualize that the medicine was brilliant little stars of light and healing that were coursing through my veins, killing all the bad stuff in my body. This practice is based on the theory that positive thoughts promote healing, that the mind-body connection is very strong. I found it very comforting.

The nurses calmly prepared me with anti-nausea medications, anti-allergic reaction medications and pain medications. The infusion took several hours. There was an extra degree of caring on their faces, and extra concern in their care. Their trips into my room were more frequent and their stays more prolonged than they might have been otherwise. They know just how dangerous these medicines can be.

For most people, the chemotherapy is toxic but not fatal. For some few people, especially those with heightened immune reactions, chemotherapy is fatal. Some months later I would read an article in an airplane magazine saying that someday, through genetic testing, physicians will be able to tell which patients should never receive certain drugs; but that technology is not yet available. In my own pretreatment education, the nurses were mindful to inform me that I was likely to feel the worst of my body's reaction to the medicine in several days.

I don't really remember my chemotherapy-birthday, but others tell me that my family visited, bearing presents and wearing heartbreaking smiles of cheer. The day was no more than a cloud to me. When I arrived home on Long Island months later, I read the cards and letters, seemingly for the first time, that had been written to me by my family and friends on that eventful fiftieth birthday.

My gratefulness for their expressions of love has helped me beyond all measure. I therefore include excerpts from their letters:

Jim wrote, "It is so difficult to express my emotions at this moment because they cover the full range that we as people are capable of. I am saddened and afraid for you as you fight to recover from this terrible illness. I can only imagine how frightening it must be for you to deal with the trauma and uncertainty of your condition. And yet you continue to amaze me with your composure, your grace and your kindness for others as you lie in your hospital bed. You are an inspiration to us all, and my love for you grows in ways I thought impossible even during this difficult time. You have been, and will always be, my one and only true love. I thank God that I found you and that He has given us such a wonderful relationship. I love you so much and will always be here for you."

From my Mom and Dad: "Our Dearest Daughter Candace – We could not find a suitable card to express our feelings for you. We find it difficult to believe how fifty years have passed. You are the most beautiful, compassionate, supportive, loving, caring person ever and you are the backbone of our family – always there for all of us when we need you. We are most happy and proud to call you our daughter. We do not know anyone who is loved by more people than you are, and you deserve that love. These have been the worst two weeks of our lives, but we now feel the burden has been lifted and that God is going to make you well again. We love you so very very much, no limits, and pray for you constantly. Thank God you have so many excellent doctors who care, most of all that you know Jesus Christ loves and cares for everything about you. We couldn't love you more."

From Brad: "Dear Mom – As I write this it is hard to make sense out of the events of the past few weeks, most of all your illness. I'm not so arrogant as to think that if God has a plan and purpose in all of this I can instantly figure it out. I've been diligently following your advice and have been praying every day and asking God for what I want. I try to remember and acknowledge all of the people out there that are suffering as badly or worse than you are, I ask for him to give you healing and the strength and courage to endure the process, I ask for the continued health and safety of Lar, Dad and the rest of the family so we can all continue to support you and finally I thank him for all the time he has given me with you up to this point. I know the past two weeks have been difficult to say the least and I know we are not out of the woods yet. I wish I could take away some of your discomfort even though I know I can't. I can reassure you that I'll be there to support you every step of the way and that I think about you whenever I am not there. I love you, Mom; I would never have come so far as a person without your constant love, support and unwavering belief in me. Happy 50th, Mom, we can beat this. Love, B."

From Lauren: "Dear Mommy – I can't begin to tell you how much you mean to me and to everyone who has been blessed enough to have you in their lives. Please know that you are in my heart, my mind and my prayers every day. Through these difficult weeks, I am reminded of the wonderful times we've had and the wonderful experiences I have had because of your love and devotion to me and Brad and Dad. Our bond will bring us through these tough times and remind us how lucky we truly are. Never forget that you can always rely on me and I that have always relied on you for strength, support, reassurance, hope and undying love. We must have faith in God's plan and patience to see it through. Love, Lar."

From our California pastor Craig and his wife Dee a verse from Philippians 2:13: "'For God is at work within you, both to will and to do of his good pleasure.' We must say, the attack on your heart still has us stunned. We know you are getting the best of care and we will continue to pray for good decisions on what to do next. We won't suggest to God how this has to happen, but our choice of course is that you rise up and walk today!"

From California church friends Don and Ann: "That there is only one you is beyond dispute. But for some reason this card reminded us of Henri Nouwen's *Prodigal Son*, 'You are my Beloved, on you my favor rests.' To be able to claim your Belovedness in the midst of recovering from this setback in your life is to affirm God's love for and control over you. We do not know what God has in store for us, but we trust in His power and goodness. We wish you complete healing and renewed strength in the weeks and months ahead. We love you both and pray for your healing and Jim's strength and your love for each other and God."

These messages of love for me – and all the caring gestures from hospital staff – were like prayers, like the finest medicine for my spirit and my body both. I know, with all my heart, that they helped me to do better.

"I would have lost heart, unless I had believed that I would see the goodness of the Lord in the land of the living." – Psalm 27:13

— ❦ —

6 THE FORSAKEN HEART

Tuesday, September 11, 2001

Brad left the hospital at 5:30 a.m. Tuesday to drive to his work in New Jersey. I was nauseated and vomiting from the chemotherapy. Jim awoke from a fitful night in his hospital chair, trying to work out the kinks in his neck and back. As is his habit, he turned on the television to watch the news. I remember watching the replay of the first plane hitting the World Trade Center, and then, with disbelief and horror, watching the second plane hit the second tower.

As the enormity of the situation began to unfold, time seemed to stand still. The staff was subdued and quiet. I overheard conversations with superiors, where they were encouraged to leave to find loved ones. As the hospital prepared for the admission of the tragedy victims, the seventeen other patients were moved out of the critical coronary care unit, my unit. My husband told me I was the only patient left; I was transported to another building via stretcher for the MUGA scan. As the stretcher was moved along the glass skyway between the two hospital buildings, people were standing silently three deep, watching the towers burn. The silence was eerie. In the testing lab no one spoke, but all went about their tasks with gentleness and deliberation. By the time I was returned to my room, the towers had collapsed.

Jim sat and watched the news coverage throughout the day. He was unable to leave the hospital, nor was my family able to visit again for several days, as all bridges, tunnels and major roadways were closed for security reasons.

Lauren was at home in California preparing for her workday, when her friend from the office called to tell her what had happened. She drove to work just so she could be near people, knowing there was no way she could call to find out how I was, much less fly home to be with me. The blackout of both information and travel was complete. She sat silently at her company staff meeting, unable to cry.

My mother was getting dressed and ready to leave her home in northern New Jersey to drive in with my wonderful Aunt Rosie. Aunt Rose called just before she left the house and told her to turn on the television. The trip was of course cancelled.

Brad was at his desk at work when word circulated through the company about what had happened. Employees were sent home, and the company along with many other companies in the New York area and across the country closed their doors.

As the morning progressed, news surfaced about the other plane crashes. The loss of life was massive; the loss of a sense of security was even greater.

As I lay there trying to comprehend what had happened to our country and to the families of the victims, I was overwhelmed by a sense of loss. Life was turned upside down – not only mine, but the whole world's. I prayed for our President, for our country, for the victims, for their families, for firemen and policemen, for the rescue workers and for the world. I was reminded of the verse that says to me, "God makes good come of all things." What good could possibly come from all this pain and suffering? As stories of heroism and courage, faith and patriotism, kindness and cohesion emerged from the headlines, God's hand became more visible.

And as I look back on this day, I am amazed at the dedication of the staff who came to work. They had to leave their families behind. They had to pass through military checkpoints at the bridges and tunnels. They had the mental and emotional wherewithal to do their work with professionalism, to show up and care for me and others in the midst of a national crisis. It was a humbling time for me.

"By humility and the fear of the Lord
are riches and honor in life." – Proverbs 22:4

———— ❤ ————

7   THE HUMBLE HEART

Later in September 2001

As I lay in my hospital bed those many weeks, I could not help but feel humbled by the resources that were being spent to prolong my life: a critical care unit bed, critical care nurses, multiple physicians, medications, medical supplies, machines, tests and so many behind-the-scenes services and service personnel. As a nurse I had some idea, though certainly not a fully accurate one, of just how much my physical care cost. I never wanted that much attention. Yet now here I was, the object of concern for so many, and so helpless to alleviate their burden of care.

I was humbled by the very intensity of this illness, by its power to disrupt our lives. It seemed as if everything stopped – time, any sense of connection to the world speeding past.

And yet, in the midst of it all, I was equally humbled by God's presence with me throughout, demonstrating his willingness to sustain me in troubled times. It has been said that when you have nothing, God is everything. How true, how true. I rested in God's hands and surrendered to His keeping.

I will never forget a sermon that was preached by the Assistant Pastor from our church in California, where she included a statement of faith, purportedly written by a martyred black South African preacher. I remember being struck by the strength of this man's faith. He must have known on some level that he was going to die and yet he does not fear; instead he appears challenged, emboldened by his situation to articulate this statement of his faith succinctly and courageously.

For me, the statement seemed the ultimate expression of humility. It went like this:

> I am part of the fellowship of the unashamed. I have the Holy Spirit power. The die has been cast. I have stepped over the line. The decision has been made – I'm a disciple of His.
>
> I won't look back, let up, slow down, be still, or back away. My past is redeemed, my present makes sense, my future is secure.
>
> I'm finished and done with low living, sight walking, smooth knees, colorless dreams, tamed visions, worldly talking, cheap giving, and dwarfed goals.
>
> I no longer need preeminence, prosperity, position, promotions, plaudits, or popularity.
>
> I don't have to be right, first, tops, recognized, praised, regarded, or rewarded.
>
> I now live by faith, lean in His presence, walk by patience, am uplifted by prayer and I labor with power.

Long ago I had printed these words and posted them on my refrigerator, where they resided for years. What comfort these words provided for me again in those uncertain times – my nation's struggle and my own. What power they reveal. By faith, we "lean in His presence."

"Pray without ceasing, in everything give thanks;
for this is the will of God in Christ Jesus for you." – Thessalonians 5:17, 18

8 THE ENLARGED HEART

Sometime in September 2001

Malcom Muggeridge wrote a book entitled *Something Beautiful for God*, about the life and works of Mother Teresa. She had heard the call to the mission field when she was only twelve years old. She never wavered in her decision to commit her life to serving God. She is purported to have said, "Love to pray, for prayer enlarges the heart until it is capable of containing God's gift of himself."

As I lay in my bed in the CCU for those many weeks, I prayed not only for myself but also in thanksgiving for all that I had been given – a generous life, a wonderful family and several church homes. I prayed for the pastors, churches and congregations that had nurtured my faith throughout the years. I tried to name all the people I knew from these churches – friends, choir directors, Sunday School teachers, Youth Group members and other kids. I tried to remember all the things we did – days at the beach, baseball games, Wednesday night dinners, Easter cantatas, Christmas caroling, visiting prisons, entertaining missionaries, Sunday night sing-along services. I realized how much I cherished these memories, how at home I had always been in church. It was a place I belonged.

I prayed "without ceasing" not only for myself, but for the other patients in the CCU as well. Despite my own dire predicament, I was aware to some degree of the suffering of the other patients. As the same family members walked past my door day after day, shoulders slumped and faces unsmiling, I knew their loved ones were in harm's way as well. Likewise, they would nod or sometimes say "God bless you" as they passed my room, offering words of support and caring.

I learned too that when another patient takes a sudden turn for the worse, you know intuitively what has happened. Hospital staff disguise the announcements with euphemistic language, but a Code Blue is not easily misunderstood. I began to pray for the other patients in the unit whom I did not know and could not see. I also prayed for their families, for comfort in their terrible time of distress and uncertainty.

The room next to mine, I smile to recall, seemed to have the greatest amount of staff activity. At all hours of the day and night, green scrub-suited staff rushed in and out. I surmised that this patient was sicker than I was and certainly in need of prayers for healing. As the weeks moved slowly by, my prayers continued for this person.

One remarkable day, my physical therapist decided I was ready to try to walk outside my room. Heretofore, I had done a few paltry steps at my bedside. Now, attached to oxygen tanks, monitors and IV poles with multiple lines, and assisted by my therapist, I made a few tentative steps outside my door. Naturally my eyes were drawn to the "patient" in the room next door, the object of my fervent prayers. Imagine my surprise when I glanced inside the room only to discover that it was the staff break room, complete with mounds of food, fresh fruit, sandwiches and beverages. I laughed right out loud! It was my first and for awhile my only guffaw.

"Every generous act of giving, with every perfect gift, is from above, coming down from the Father." – James 1:17

———— ❤ ————

9   ROOM IN MY HEART

"Things aren't always what they seem. Every now and then something happens that challenges us to see other people or perhaps ourselves in a new light. That challenge forces us to reconsider long held beliefs and see the world from a new perspective."

– The Rev. Dr. Charles Cary

Sometime in September 2001

About three weeks into my stay in the CCU at NYPH/C, the physicians made the decision to attempt to move me out to the general medical floor. I suspect that the decision reflected pressure from internal hospital authorities or policies, regarding length of stay in the unit. Reluctantly, my physicians gave the order to titrate down the intravenous medicines that supported my blood pressure. My dose was already very small, the doctor explained, and probably didn't really have much of an effect anyway. So over the next several hours the dose would be gradually decreased until it was turned off, and then I would be moved out to the floor.

It had now been about five or six weeks that I had been a patient in the critical care areas of several hospitals. The thought of moving out to the floor – away from the watchful eyes of the kindly ever-vigilant, ubiquitous, highly skilled nurses with whom I did not need to communicate with words – was frightening to say the least. As the nurses readied me for departure, I became more and more depressed. I knew I wasn't well enough to be independent, to use the bathroom on my own or to walk on my own. Almost everything had been done for me. And though I tried never to be a problem to the nurses, to use my call bell incessantly or make unnecessary requests, the bottom line was that I needed them. As the staff wheeled me out of my room before dinner, Jim walking alongside, I could not hold back my tears. I was leaving a protective environment of caring, attentive individuals for the floor: no place for the faint of heart.

As we headed down the hall to my new room, the first thing I noticed was how far it was from the nurses' station. I was assigned to a two-bed room, the other bed already occupied by an apparently sleeping patient who was attended by a uniformed member of the hospital staff, sitting in a chair at the foot of the bed. I would come to understand that she was a babysitter for the sleeping patient who had a tendency to wander when she became confused. The room was small, crowded with people and equipment and dimly lit. The television was loud, blaring the repetitive Looney Tunes medley after each two-minute cartoon. I had missed dinner in the transition, so Jim ran out to get me something to eat, but I was too exhausted to eat it. Once I was settled with my own television and telephone, Jim said goodnight and left for home at about 7 p.m. He was no happier than I was at the new turn of events.

Finally, about 10 p.m. I asked the sleeping patient's attendant if she would mind turning down the television. She replied, "I'm not watching television," and made no attempt to adjust the volume. Her tone was hostile. The refusal to comply with my request was both surprising and unexpected. I was dismayed. For no reason I could determine, this person had decided to make things difficult for me. I felt so terrible and so helpless. The noise was loud and unremitting. I was distraught from fatigue and poor health. What was happening?

I struggled to my feet, grabbed on to my IV pole for support and shuffled out to the floor to find my nurse. The floor nurses came and asked the attendant to turn down the television. A minor adjustment was made in the volume, but not enough to make a difference. I was in for a long night.

Alternately I dozed, only to be awakened repeatedly by glaring overhead lights each time one of the attendant's friends came in to have a conversation with her. I wept silently in my bed. Miraculously, the patient would sleep from the time of my arrival until the next morning, undisturbed. But the TV stayed on.

Finally, at about 2 a.m., I got up, grabbed the IV pole again and dragged myself to the waiting room where I sat in a chair for the rest of the night until just before the doctor came in the next morning. The nurses were upset too, but no other beds were available on the unit and I was adamant that I felt better in the quiet of the waiting room.

I prayed and I cried. I was feeling very sorry for myself. I had been trying to do something good in going to Africa to do something about AIDS. Now I found myself suffering alone, completely without the emotional resources or physical reserves to deal with any of it.

As I prayed, the hands on the clock moved slowly. I opened my eyes and watched the lights on the George Washington Bridge. The bridge looks to be made of fine crystal when it is all lit up. On this night, only some of the lights were on as the terrorist threats of bridge bombings were still looming. A huge American flag waved lazily in a gentle breeze. It really was quite beautiful. For a time a kind of peace settled over me. I was vulnerable and powerless and in physical pain, but at least I was alive.

The doctor came in very early to check on me. He appeared horrified to know that I had spent most of the night in the waiting room chair. The child in me replied with indignation, "How could you do this to me?" In conversation with his colleagues, he came to the conclusion that I could not tolerate being off blood pressure medication, which meant that I had to be transferred back to the CCU. I saw this move as a failure, as a sign that in fact I was not getting better, and might not ever come out of the hospital alive. His nurse practitioner tried to explain that I would feel better once the vasopressor medication was restarted. She also ordered a psychiatric consult.

Clearly, I *was* depressed. Back in my room, the psychiatrist arrived, drawing the curtain between us and my roommates. I told the psychiatrist about how my life had turned upside down in the last five weeks. I told her I had been a healthy, active wife and mother one day and critically ill the next. I told her how I was moved between three hospitals and how I had almost died three times. I poured out my heart, my tears and my pain. I was not sure I would ever go home. I painstakingly went through every detail.

She listened carefully, offered anti-depressant medication and left to consult with my doctors. My issues were real life and death issues and she did appear to understand that. There wasn't really anything she could say otherwise, so at least she didn't trivialize it, which I appreciated. I was grateful for her visit and the feeling that she had at least listened. Medication wasn't going to help me, however, because my issues were spiritual ones. I needed to put my faith in order.

When the curtain was opened again, the hostile attendant was in the process of leaving her post and her charge to the care of the day shift. The patient was sitting up in bed eating breakfast. She was a young woman, of Latino descent. She did not speak English. The kitchen staff delivered my tray. It had a variety of things that I had not ordered, that per doctor's orders I could not eat, including hard-boiled egg, caffeinated coffee, Danish.

I must have stared at the tray in dismay and started to cry again. I was starving and yet again wasn't going to eat. The lovely young lady started handing me food from her own tray. With eyes filled with compassion and understanding, she tried to comfort me, to reach out to me in my distress. Having slept she was oblivious to all that had happened the night before. But despite the language barrier and her own physical limitations, she read my distress loud and clear and didn't hesitate to try to help. I remember her kindness still. She was an angel in disguise.

With her sweetness juxtaposed against the treatment from her night attendant, I couldn't help but see the irony in my treatment from the two individuals. All the while I felt so alone, God was with me. His love poured out from the patient in the next bed. Within the hour I was returned to CCU by stretcher and restarted on the vasopressor medications – a huge step backwards, but it was where I felt safe.

Sometime in the weeks that followed the vasopressor drugs were turned off again and I was moved out of CCU a second time – now to a private room on the general medical floor. I was more comfortable with this change, perhaps because I finally didn't need the vasopressor drugs. The move came shortly after lunch, just in time to have monitors in place and a telephone turned on in my room so I could make some calls to family and friends.

Before long, however, several members of the nursing staff came rushing into my room – one taking my blood pressure, another hooking me up to a portable defibrillator, a third asking direct questions: Did I feel okay? Did I have any pain? Was I dizzy? On their heels came Dr. Deborah Ascheim – another wonderful heart failure cardiologist, who subsequently would become my cardiac biopsy doctor.

Dr. Ascheim is tall, beautiful, extremely bright and just as kind. She explained calmly that monitors showed I was in a slow, life-threatening heart rhythm that was not responding to the intravenous medications she had ordered to stop it, so I needed to go back to CCU. Apparently my heart was so badly scarred that it simply could not beat correctly. Dr. Ascheim ran alongside my bed while the nurses raced me through the corridors to the safety of the CCU.

Back in the CCU unit the nurses offered me my old room, with the gorgeous view of the Hudson River. Within ten minutes of my return the life-threatening rhythm broke. They didn't try to move me out a third time. I would meet Dr. Ascheim again not long after the transplant. She would become an important part of my life.

♥

"As I prayed, the hands on the clock moved slowly. I opened my eyes and watched the lights on the George Washington Bridge. The bridge looks to be made of fine crystal when it is all lit up. . . ."

———————————————————————

*"Blessed are those who hunger and thirst for righteousness' sake,
for they shall be filled." –* Matthew 5:6

— ♥ —

10 THE HUNGRY HEART

Sometime in September 2001

Clearly, the only thing NewYork-Presbyterian didn't do especially well was food service! (A universal hospital observation, I know . . .) The Dietary Department handed out menus a day ahead. You were given at least two choices for each category on the menu, like an appetizer of soup or salad, a main course beef stew or tuna fish salad, fresh fruit or jello for dessert. A patient's particular diet is determined by his doctor; no choices there. All heart patients are put on a low salt, low cholesterol and calorie-restricted diet. If they happen to have a problem with sugar, then they are placed on a diabetic diet. When you're a patient in a hospital, two things happen; time stands still and you lose control over everything. Illness takes away most of your control over your life, hospitalization takes away the rest.

Of necessity, the hospital functions on its own time clock and that revolves around meals. Truly, other than visits from your family, you feel you have almost nothing to look forward to. Sometimes patients are so sick they don't even look forward to visits. Not because they don't love their families, but because it's simply too much effort physically and emotionally to participate in conversation. Visitors are in the world, you are not. They can come and go, you cannot. They can take a shower, eat whatever and whenever they want, talk on the phone, drive a car, feel the sunshine on their face and avoid pain; you cannot. The only thing you do have to look forward to is meals. And even meals get cancelled if you have to have an empty stomach for a scheduled test, or you just happen to miss the meal because you were having a procedure in some other part of the hospital.

So, despite the fact that you don't necessarily feel like eating anyway, you do anticipate the moment of seeing your selections brought to you on a tray. It's much more than simply dining; there's a small but important element of control. When what you ordered doesn't come on the tray, the one "bright spot" of your day, you feel betrayed, defeated.

All three meals in NYPH/C and most hospitals are served within one eight-hour shift. Breakfast is at 9 a.m. Lunch is at 1 p.m. and dinner is at 5 p.m. As a giant cell patient I was taking highly toxic medications at intervals during all waking hours, from 6 a.m. up until bedtime at 10 p.m.; most have to be taken with food and/or fluids. I also had food restrictions that limited what might safely appear on my tray.

Heart failure patients are restricted to a 2 gram sodium, low-fluid diet. A normal person eats approximately 4-20 grams of sodium per day. Heart failure patients have a tendency to retain fluid in the vascular tree, which causes more work for the heart. By removing table salt and salt in cooking you can significantly reduce salt intake, and hope to preserve some heart function. The food is tasteless but that's beside the point. It's an essential restriction.

Most natural foods intrinsically have a small amount of sodium in them. For heart failure patients, I found, a sample menu for the next day is passed out with your breakfast tray as it is for all other patients in the hospital. I put a great deal of deliberation and effort into making my selections, despite what tempting delicacies appeared on the list of choices. However, the dieticians of course review the menu choices made by the heart failure patients and adjust what actually gets sent on the patient's tray, depending on sodium and calorie content. So, at mealtime you expect to receive what you have chosen and what actually comes is oftentimes something different and considerably less. I swear it was some sort of a test for mental toughness! And of all the battles I fought each day to stay alive, this one almost beat me.

One night for dinner I got a one-cup portion of boiled rice; that's all. That's it. Here I was with monitors and tubes and a million devices, it seems, and my much-anticipated meal was . . . rice. The dietician had apparently calculated my sodium intake and/or calorie intake for the day and figured I had exceeded my limits. What she didn't know was that I hadn't eaten any of it! Heart failure patients do sometimes harbor the misconception that their portions are cut in half, and it did seem to be so for me. I found out later that my portions were exactly what they should have been.

♥

"When you're a patient in a hospital, two things happen; time stands still and you lose control over everything. Illness takes away most of your control over your life, hospitalization takes away the rest. . . ."

"Sometimes patients are so sick they don't even look forward to visits. . . .
Visitors are in the world, you are not. They can come and go, you cannot.
They can take a shower, eat whatever and whenever they want, talk on the
phone, drive a car, feel the sunshine on their face and avoid pain; you cannot.
The only thing you do have to look forward to is meals. . . ."

"For He shall give His angels charge over you
to keep you in all your ways." – Psalm 91:11

11 ROOMMATES

Sometime in September 2001

My earliest memory as a child is one in which I am about eighteen months old. I am lying on the cold hardwood floor of my darkened room at night, on my stomach, peering under the door, trying to be near the light peeking in under the door. My parents said I used to hate to go to bed at night. They would put me in my crib and let me howl until I fell asleep. When it got quiet they would slowly open the door to my room, gently pushing my little body out of the way and then settling me back in my crib. Even way back then, I didn't like to be alone.

My sister Mare was born when I was three and a half years old. From then on, she was my roommate. I loved having a roommate. Just knowing that she was there made me comfortable. Though we're very different people, we have always been extremely close. She played with toys; I played with people. She was shy; I was outgoing. As we grew up, she was tall and skinny; I was short and plump. She was "crafty" – liked doing things with her hands; I loved to cook. We were both athletic, but I liked team sports and she liked individual sports.

No matter the differences between us, however, Mare and I were and are much more than sisters. She is my friend, my confidante. Sometimes I am her mother and sometimes she is mine.

When I married Jim at the age of twenty, he became my next roommate. And now, so many years and so many shared memories later, my illness changed everything – as well as I thought I knew Jim and he me, our words are even kinder. The thoughts we share are deeper. Our respect for each other is palpable. In my recovery, no request was denied. No "please would you" was too much trouble or at a bad time. Nothing was too trivial, too much effort or inconvenient. Jim left for work every day with a sense of guilt and uncertainty. Would I be happy or worse? Would I be okay? I tried to be as little trouble as possible. With regard to the house, as we learned, nothing really has to be done urgently. Everything can be postponed. Little things don't matter.

As the month of September 2001 waned, my heart deteriorated still further. I was failing day by day and I knew it. I lay in my bed in CCU wondering if I would ever feel the warmth of sunshine on my skin or a gentle breeze on my face. I thought, so this is what it's like to be dying. I didn't expect it to happen so soon. I had planned my daughter's wedding in my mind. I longed for grandchildren. When we tried unsuccessfully to have more children in our late thirties, I set my sights instead on the children of my children. My husband and I had often discussed retirement plans and destinations. I fully expected to grow old with him.

I studied my family each day, savoring the mere sight of them, their voices, their mannerisms, the color of their eyes, the cowlicks in their hair, wondering . . . was today the last day I would see them? Curiously, I did not live those days in fear. I knew God was with me. I did, however, live those days in grief. Had I told my children enough times that I loved them? Had I made my husband happy?

Months later, Jim told me that during that bleak time he was formulating my eulogy in his mind. And in fact at the same time I was thinking about my own eulogy, the resume of my life. Had I done enough? Had I lived my life well? Had I treasured every moment? To be honest, no, I had not. I saw myself as always struggling, impatient, trying too hard, giving too much, not taking care of myself, not forgiving myself my shortcomings. Quick with a sharp word or snap judgment. No, I had clearly failed, but the beauty of being a Christian is not that we become perfect, but that we are forgiven each transgression and no matter what, we are loved.

In the solitude of my room in the middle of the night I lay exhausted, alone and dying. One of my nurses came in to ask in a gentle voice if she could do anything to make me more comfortable. I asked her if there was any way that I could turn to lie on my side. Given all the tubes and devices that was not easily accomplished, but we managed. I grasped the bed rail to stabilize my position. She then left me alone.

Such a small kind of assistance, but it meant so much to me. I watched the vehicles travel up and down the West Side Highway, wondering if the occupants knew how lucky they were to be driving a car, going someplace, free to work or play. My heart was heavy but grateful for the nurse's earlier help. I drifted in and out of consciousness.

At some point, I became aware that someone was holding my hand. The grasp was light but firm, warm and comforting. The hand enveloped mine. I did not open my eyes. I thought it was one of the nurses. I was grateful for the company. I let myself relax and I fell into a deep sleep.

When I awakened some time later, my first awareness was of the hand still holding mine. When I opened my eyes, no one was there. At first I was surprised, then I was not surprised, but pleased as the awareness of God's presence washed over me. The brief respite from suffering allowed me to hang on a little longer. God seemed to say, could you do this for me?

"I lay in my bed in CCU wondering if I would ever feel the warmth of sunshine on my skin or a gentle breeze on my face. I thought, so this is what it's like to be dying. I didn't expect it to happen so soon. . . ."

"You have granted me life and favor,
and Your care has preserved my spirit." – Job 10:12

— ♥ —

12 THE GIFT OF LIFE

Saturday, September 29, 2001

Though I didn't realize it at the time, today was the day my flight with the Save the Children group was scheduled to leave for Malawi. Anne Lawlor, the medical social worker for inpatients of the Heart Failure Team, dropped in to see me on Friday morning before the weekly meeting of the forty-member heart failure team. My case was on the agenda for discussion that day just as it had been each Friday since my admission to NewYork-Presbyterian four weeks before.

When the treatment plan was laid out at the time I was admitted, it called for me to receive three treatments of Cytoxan, an intravenous chemotherapy, three weeks apart. At the end of the nine weeks I was to be reevaluated and if necessary placed on the active transplant list. If successful, that treatment plan would have put me home in time for Christmas.

I had received only one treatment three weeks before and today I was scheduled to receive the second. But it wasn't working. I was failing fast and I knew it. I had been for a MUGA scan the day before and though the doctors did not give me hard numbers, they did say that the results were not good. They looked somber and sad in relaying the information to me.

My cousin Jan came to visit that day and brought lunch – a turkey sandwich made by her mother, my Aunt Rose. I was sitting in the chair in my room. I was so exhausted I couldn't hold my head up. I had no energy even to smile, much less talk to my cousin whom I love. Normally, a homemade turkey sandwich, especially one from my aunt who is a great cook, would have perked me up a bit. But that day, no.

I told Anne Lawler that I was ready for the transplant, that I knew I was failing and that I had had enough suffering. She had tears in her eyes. She promised to convey my feelings to the committee.

That afternoon, Dr. Deng came to see me. He was excited. He said that based on the information Anne passed on to the team that morning, and in the ensuing discussion, the decision had been made to place me on the active transplant list. Now the wait would begin. Projected waiting time was weeks to months. I knew I would not live that long. Best-case scenario – a heart almost immediately available, and a miracle in itself – would get me out of the hospital for Christmas. I wasn't sure that emotionally I could cope with that timeline. But of course I didn't have the choice.

Sunday, September 30

I had been supposed to receive the second intravenous Cytoxan on Friday, but there was a problem with the PIC line in my right arm. It was a two-lumen line and one of the lumens was occluded by a blood clot. I needed both lines, as I was again dependent on the intravenous medicines that maintained my blood pressure.

The PIC line nurse had injected an anticoagulant, or "clot buster," into the line early Friday morning, to try to dissolve the clot. Four hours later she came back to flush the line and it did not open up. The chemo was delayed.

It was Friday night, well after quitting time, when the head nurse of the PIC line department, Randy, showed up in my room. He did not go home to his family because he knew that I needed the chemo and I couldn't receive it until the line was open. The PIC line had to work. Randy patiently, painstakingly and gently manipulated the anticoagulant solution in and out of the port in my arm, each time letting it sit for an extended period, giving it time to work. It is time-intensive, this process, because if it is hurried, a clot can be dislodged and travel to the lungs or brain, causing death. Well into the evening hours the line finally opened. I will always treasure Randy's care of me.

I got the chemotherapy with my son Brad at my bedside. Jim was home with a respiratory infection, on antibiotics. As he was infectious and I was immuno-suppressed, he could not be with me. I missed him terribly, but was so thankful to have my son. At the same time, it broke my heart to see him. There was so much pain in his face. He hadn't slept well in over a month. He'd lost weight, was pale and obviously depressed and in emotional shock. Surely, there are many victims in every tragedy – the person to whom the tragedy occurs, and the family who loves yet has to watch the suffering.

Prior to this whole experience, our children had never entertained the thought that Jim or I might die. Our family discussions about death centered on their aging grandparents, who have always been a huge influence in their lives. Lauren told me later that the entire extended family fell apart in sadness with my illness. She said I was always the one who handled any family crisis, rushing to everyone's bedside to provide comfort and support. She said that with *me* as the patient, their efforts to care for me and for each other were disorganized and somehow not enough.

Lauren is my verbal child, the one with deep emotions who can put into words what her heart is feeling. Brad is also a very feeling person, yet he stores his feelings deep inside. On this bedside visit, the pain on his face was terrible to see. It broke *my* heart.

Transplant Day – Monday, October 1

Again, though I realized it only later, today my Save the Children group had been scheduled to land in Malawi, and that due to the events of 9/11 the flight was cancelled.

The nurses came into my room at one o'clock in the morning on October 1st with astounding news: miraculously – just two days after Dr. Deng's visit – my new heart was on the way and I was on the operating room schedule for 6 a.m. Never for a minute, knowing the usual weeks-to-months wait for hearts, had I dared to hope for this – two days, not even a half of one week. But it was happening.

I had suffered greatly, not knowing from day to day or even from minute to minute whether I would live or die. The Bible says to tell God exactly what you want, in prayer, for He can provide more than we can ask or even think. My sister Mare is living proof of answered prayer. She is a Stage IV breast cancer survivor of fifteen years. With incredible courage and faith, she has climbed mountains all over the world – literally and figuratively – inspiring cancer victims to have hope in the face of such a terrible diagnosis. She's been on television programs and in television documentaries. She travels across the country speaking on behalf of the Breast Cancer Fund, which raises money for breast cancer research and treatment. Today Mare radiates life and health. She would never entertain the thought that I would not get well. She simply wouldn't hear of it. The ultimate possibility thinker.

Repeatedly over the past months, I had told God I did not want to climb mountains, accomplish great things or become famous. I just wanted to go home. The possibility of a new heart gave me the first opportunity in two months to entertain the thought that I might live. My first reaction was ineffable joy. I cried. The reaction was swiftly followed but yet another powerful reaction – grief for the family of the donor who was at this moment suffering just like me. What a courageous decision to make in the midst of so much pain.

John Landers, a heart transplant recipient ten years ago, expresses this dichotomy of feelings well in the publication *Transplant Chronicles:* "People come to the point of heart transplantation from one of two clinical scenarios. Either the patient has struggled with illness for much of their lives and the possibility of end stage organ failure has always been the ultimate outcome. [Or], some of us became sick so fast, we did not have a chance to prepare in any way for the answer to end stage organ failure. The answer, 'You need a transplant in order to save your life' and the gravity of that statement simply stuns us and leaves us reeling out of control. Why me? What are my chances? Will it work? What kind of life will I have? How much time do I have? We fight hard to live, sometimes right on the edge of death, while we wait for a donor. Though we want so much to live, the thought of someone else dying and saving our lives via donation is troubling. We recognize this rationally as possible, but it is again something that leaves us feeling remorse. Someone's loved one will die and because that person chose at the height of grief to donate, we receive the greatest gift, a second chance."

There are fortunately guidelines by which a transplant recipient can write an anonymous letter to the donor family. It is so hard to put these feelings into words. You want so much to tell them how grateful you are, and yet how sad you are for their loss. Though I did not want to know about the donor at the time, I knew as a former ICU nurse that organ donors are often young people who have died as a result of trauma, such as a car accident. The parents have experienced a sudden, unexpected, overwhelming tragedy. In the midst of their pain they make a courageous decision. As a recipient, you will benefit and eventually get better. Yet their suffering will last a lifetime.

The Heart Transplant team at NYPH/C, under the auspices of Drs. Niloo Edwards and Donna Mancini, has prepared a manual with all kinds of valuable information for the heart transplant patient: *The Patient's Guide to Heart*

Transplantation at New York-Presbyterian. When first admitted and considered a candidate for the transplant list I was given a copy of this manual. I was so sick that I hadn't had the strength to hold the book or the energy to read it. Yet I've read it many times since October 1 – my transplant day – and still refer to it on a regular basis. It's an excellent resource.

Among other things, the booklet contains the history of heart transplantation. In 1967, Dr. Christiaan Barnard from Cape Town, South Africa, transplanted the heart of a twenty-five-year-old woman into the chest of a fifty-five-year-old man dying of heart damage. Miraculously, the man lived for eighteen days.

Over the next twenty years, important advances took place in the areas of tissue typing and immunosuppressive drugs, which allowed more transplant operations and markedly improved patient survival rates. New York-Presbyterian's first cardiac transplant was performed in 1977. It was the third medical institution in the entire country to perform heart transplants. Cyclosporine was approved by the FDA for commercial use in 1983, and is still the most commonly prescribed immunosuppressive drug in organ transplantation today. Research has continued steadily in the areas of immunosuppression, infection control and temporary and permanent mechanical heart devices. All of these advances have contributed to the improved outlook for patients with end stage cardiac disease.

Another book I would later read – *Organ Transplantation*, by Frank P. Stuart, Michael M. Abecassis and Dixon B. Kaufman – told me still more about transplantation and the extraordinary good fortune of my own experience. There are presently one hundred heart transplant centers throughout the country, two-hundred fifty centers for kidney, twenty-five centers for lung and fifteen centers for intestine. Many physicians and surgeons have now been trained. Nevertheless, people die every single day while waiting for an organ. There is huge disparity between the number of patients waiting for new organs and the number of organs that actually become available. The waiting list for all organs is, as noted, approaching 85,000 individuals; yet the number of cadaver donors has stalled at approximately 5,000 each year. Because supply and demand are so far out of balance, consensus on fairness in allocation is difficult to achieve.

My own experience had to follow important established guidelines. Since 1984, the NYPH/C manual notes, UNOS, the United Network for Organ Sharing, has held a federal contract to oversee the national organ sharing system. It is a complicated system that coordinates all aspects of organ donation – from public and professional education, donor evaluation, family counseling and consent, medical management of the donor, maximum recovery of all usable organs and organ preservation, to distribution and transportation, follow-up and reporting. The system deals with diverse medical, ethical, political and regulatory issues, all while under intense public scrutiny. UNOS's declared purpose is to promote and advance the science of transplantation, and to increase the availability of donor organs. It manages a national computer database with a waiting list that matches donor organs to recipients as fairly as possible, without regard for gender, race, religion, lifestyle and financial or social status.

Donor hearts are provided to patients based on the donor's blood type and body weight, I learned from the NYPH/C manual, as well as on the recipient's severity of illness and geographic location. A suitable donor is a young to middle-aged person who has been declared "brain dead" based on standard criteria, and whose heart is still functioning. All donors are screened for the presence of hepatitis and HIV infections. Any evidence of these infections precludes use of the organ for transplantation. When a transplant team is notified of the availability of a suitable heart, they travel quickly to the donor hospital to prepare the heart for transportation. They must move quickly as the donor heart can be disconnected from a person's circulation for only about four hours before it loses its ability to work properly when reconnected within the transplant recipient.

The wise NewYork-Presbyterian nurses had warned me that it was possible I would wake up in the Recovery Room without a new heart. The patient is prepared for surgery, placed under anesthesia, the chest may be opened – and then the heart surgeon may decide that the organ is just not right. This can even happen more than once. Thankfully, this did not happen to me.

It was time to get ready for my transplant surgery. When I was in CCU all those weeks, my cousin Jan brought me a tape of a Unity Church service in which she sang a solo, her first ever. She wanted me to hear it. She had been taking voice lessons. I listened to that tape literally a hundred times during my hospitalization. I knew all the songs by heart. One of them was, "I'm Living in the Light of the Lord." I still sing it all the time.

It just so happens that the tape was from the first Sunday following the World Trade Center collapses – by which time I had been in various hospitals for nearly a month. The sermon had to do with why God let the tragedy occur. The total lack of security on the world scene so closely paralleled the utter lack of control and security I was feeling just before surgery, that hearing the tape lent comfort to me.

When they woke me up at 1 a.m. on that October 1st to say I was on the schedule that morning for 6 a.m. to get my new heart, I was grateful and at the same time grief-stricken. Grief-stricken for myself, for my family, for the donor family and for the country. It was too much suffering. I imagined that my donor was probably a teenager. I found out later that was so.

As an Intensive Care Unit nurse I had been through this many times. I had cared for dying children and comforted grieving parents. I would pray with them and for them. As a nurse, you never walk away from those situations untouched. You carry them with you in your heart forever. I would go home at night and give my own children an extra hug.

The nurses immediately brought me a portable phone so I could call Jim and have him come in to be with me before the surgery. Because he had been sick, I hadn't seen him for five days. The nurses said he could wear a mask, but it was really important that he come. Brad had just left my bedside several hours before. I used the phone to call the Unity Church 800 number, a twenty-four-hour prayer line, and someone prayed with me. While I waited for Jim to arrive, I put Jan's tape on again. It was such a comfort to feel I was in the middle of a worship service, surrounded by what had become a familiar and loving congregation, listening to wonderful music and feeling God's presence in the midst of it all.

The staff was bustling around now, efficiently weighing and measuring and generally prepping me for surgery. They asked what I was listening to. I told them it was a tape of a sermon. I could see they were glad that it brought me such great comfort. Their attitude enhanced that sense of comfort.

Months later, I wrote a letter to the pastor of Jan's church and told him what strength I had derived from that often-played sermon tape. In a critical care area, you have nothing of your own: no jewelry, not a stitch of clothing, nothing that belongs to you. You are stripped down to your birthday suit. I didn't even have a Bible, but then I didn't have the energy to hold one or the powers of concentration to read it. The room is filled instead with equipment and gadgets that are necessary to monitor you, and emergency equipment to keep you alive. This tape, however, was my lifeline. It was one of many blessings, one of the many ways that God cared for me and made His presence known to me in my darkest hour.

When Jim arrived at 3 a.m., we started calling family. By 5 a.m. Brad and my sister Mare and her husband had arrived at my bedside. Lauren, in California, had sent her dearest love to me and called the airlines immediately to arrange a flight. My brother Sam told me later that he thought Jim was calling to tell him I had died. He had been awake, thinking about me.

The nurses cautiously explained to my family, as they had to me, that it was possible I could wake up with an incision but without a new heart, that sometimes after surgery has begun and the chest is open, the physicians determine that the heart is not right. Perhaps not the right fit. Apparently, the weighing and measuring is important. I was five foot four and weighed a hundred and fifty pounds – at least twenty pounds lighter than when this whole thing had started six weeks before, on August 17. Another one of the many blessings for me that day: not just the availability of the heart, but the perfect fit. And many more blessings would follow.

The following is a poem written to me soon after the surgery by our dear friend Dan Holland, from our former church in Trabuco Canyon, California. Dan wrote, "Though a continent may separate us, you need to know how fervently all of us back here are praying for you and Jim. We still feel your presence."

I Have a New Heart

This here life is plumb exhausting;
It wears me to the bone.
Sometimes I wish my Savior
Would just up and call me home.
But then I hear the whippoorwill,
Or see the harvest moon;
So I tell the Lord, "if you call me,
Don't make it quite so soon."

I have a new heart
And it's filled with Jesus Christ.
I have a new heart,
And I celebrate His life.
I have a new heart;
Lord, let me spread your love.
I have a new heart,
And it came from God above.

Enduring trials, they tell me,
Build my character and soul.
I can only climb the ladder
From the bottom of the hole.
Tough lessons, to be sure,
My Redeemer did impart.
But they helped me realize
I have a brand new heart.

I have a new heart,
And it's filled with Jesus Christ.
I have a new heart,
And I celebrate His life.
I have a new heart;
Lord, let me spread Your love.
I have a new heart,
And it came from God above.

My tender, tender Father
Will always lend a helping hand.
He would never, ever make me
Go through more than I could stand.
And when He finally calls me
To the new life I will start,
I'll hop aboard the golden train
With a brand new heart.

I have a new heart,
And it's filled with Jesus Christ.
I have a new heart,
And I celebrate His life.
I have a new heart;
Lord, let me spread your love.
I have a new heart,
And it came from God above.

Weeks later on December 4, home and recovering well, I would read the letter and the poem for the first time. I was deeply moved and wrote Dan to tell him so –

"Dearest Dan: Jim saved all the cards and letters that we received while I was in the hospital. He would read them to me when he arrived in the evening and we would cry together, so grateful were we for the deep sense of God's grace that was expressed in each one. . . ."

I told Dan too that a retired pastor who is unknown to me but is a treasured friend of my parents called to see how I was doing when I was staying at my parents' house following my discharge from the hospital. When I told him I was improving, he said, "Legions of angels are rejoicing on your behalf!" Such a beautiful image.

And I told Dan that before and after the surgery, still other unbelievable blessings were tied up in the day-to-day struggle for my life. The doctors and the nurses cared for me, prayed for me and prayed with me. They put their arms around me and cried with me. I never could have survived without this dimension of their care. It's something that could never be legally requested in a job description, but, oh, what a difference it made to me. It was almost as if God, like the director of a movie, had placed each of them there to demonstrate His love for me and reassure me with His presence.

On the morning of the transplant, it meant the world to me to have my family present and praying for me, whether down the hall or across the country.

When I arrived in the Operating Room my anesthesiologist explained that he needed to insert two new arterial lines. He required two new patent lines in the event that I needed emergency medication or blood during surgery. Without local anesthesia, just as before, he tried several times to insert a line in my right wrist. Frustrated and apologetic with his lack of success, he called for assistance. Two new doctors attempted to insert arterial lines in my left arm, again without local anesthesia. Time was running out, because of the narrow window during which the organ is still viable before it starts to break down, and then can no longer be used. The doctors all apologized profusely for hurting me. I knew that with me in failure and with no peripheral pulse, locating an artery was all but impossible.

This process seemed to go on forever, with pain that brought me to tears, and then finally, finally, success. I glanced at the clock. It was 8 a.m. That's the last thing I remember.

Apparently, by that time, my entire family was in the waiting room with the exception of course of Lauren, who was taking an early morning flight out of San Jose. The wait must have been so hard for them all. Several anxious hours later Dr. Deng came out to say that everything had gone well and my new heart was "perfect." His manner conveyed the extraordinary care and concern of the whole transplant team. My family expressed their joy with hugs and grateful tears all around.

I was soon transferred to the post-transplant intensive care. Like CCU, it was a private room. My nurse sat on a stool at my bedside and never left the room. I was on a respirator with a tube down my throat and unable to talk. Jim says that the family visited my bedside throughout the day and that I made eye contact, but I don't remember anything at all. My first conscious thought, which was about 10 o'clock that night, was of Jim coming through the door of my room and saying, "Look at the present Brad brought for you!" Brad had just picked up his cargo at Kennedy Airport. It was my beautiful daughter Lauren. I remember her radiant smile and the brilliant light that surrounded her face. I was alive! She tells me I tried to mouth "Sunshine" to her. My second conscious thought was that I felt wonderful, tubes, IV's, stitches and all, I felt absolutely wonderful!

As I became more alert, waking the next morning, I started to fight the endotracheal tube. I felt as if I were choking and I couldn't breathe. My nurse called for back-up and a set of wrist restraints, lest I pull the tube out prematurely. I gestured by moving my fingers in a circular motion, as though I were writing, that I wanted to say something on a piece of paper. I was not confused, I was not going to pull out the tube. I wanted to tell them that the tube had a kink in it and I was not getting the air I needed. What the nurses saw as confusion was in fact panic. I needed to tell them what was really happening. They swiftly handed me a clipboard, and I could tell them what was wrong.

The nurses calmly instructed me to breathe around the tube, which I had not known I could do. They explained carefully that they had to test my blood oxygen level, and if it was okay they would contact the doctor and get permission to remove the tube. Everyone had to be sure I could breathe on my own before they could remove it. After what seemed like an eternity, it was removed. Thank goodness for the clipboard.

When Jim and the kids came into my room on what I think was the next morning, I was sitting up in bed alternately sipping ginger ale and vomiting. This was now day two following my second chemo treatment, and this was the day the nausea sets in. What an amazing coinciding of events: nausea from treatment for the old heart, which had just been replaced by a new one!

Between bouts of regurgitation, though, I was beaming. My daughter laughed at me. My dear husband who had probably been up for more than forty-eight hours turned green and almost passed out. The nurses rushed to get him to a chair so he wouldn't get hurt if he went down. It was all too much for him. He hadn't eaten, he hadn't slept and here I was with a huge incision down my chest and two chest tubes. We joked about making room for him in my bed.

13 OCTOBER 1, 2001 . . . TRANSPLANT DAY:
A SON'S PERSPECTIVE

I'd left Mom at midnight. I sat with her as she received the last of her second round of chemotherapy. She looked so little in the bed. She had lost so much weight. The chemo seemed to weigh her down. She kissed me good-bye and said for the thousandth time that she loved me, no matter what.

My body was beyond tired. I hadn't eaten or slept much over the past six weeks. I no longer knew what it was like to feel normal. I'd lost weight. My stomach was in shreds. At all hours I would call my sister in California to talk, but nothing helped and nothing changed the fact that Mom was dying. I didn't want to be here. I did not want Mom to be in this situation. But there wasn't anything I could do to change it. I just couldn't imagine my life without her. But here I was. Desperate measures had to be taken in desperate times. And the transplant was one of them.

After working the full day I commuted into the City to be with her because Dad was sick and I didn't want her to be alone. She was really sick – it was hard to tell the difference at this point between fatigue, heart failure and depression. She'd gone almost ten rounds and was down for the count and she knew it. Time was running out. She was encouraged because she had just been placed 1A on the UNOS transplant list (United Network of Organ Sharing), but equally subdued with the knowledge that someone had to die in order for her to live. She didn't talk much. She was too weak. She really missed Dad.

I drove to my G'parents' house because I didn't want to be alone. I slept there briefly until my cell phone rang at 2 a.m. It was Dad. Mom's new heart was on the way and the nurses wanted the family to come right now to be with her. Dad sounded frightened and excited both at the same time. I didn't know what to feel. I was so tired that I felt sick.

I showered and dressed and waited for Aunt Mare and John to arrive so we could all drive back to the City. I parked on the street to save money, arriving about 4 a.m. Dad was at her side with a mask on to protect Mom from getting his cold. Mom was on the operating room schedule for 6 a.m. She burst into tears when she saw me. Up to this point every single thing had gone wrong in our family every day for the last six weeks. I was afraid to hope and terrified not to.

The nurses brought Mom the phone so she could call her parents. The nurses were all excited for Mom. They bustled around her bed, darting in and out of the room rustling pieces of paper, equipment and medications.

Somewhere around 7 a.m. she left. We walked alongside the stretcher as long as we could until she disappeared inside the OR doors. We stood there together stunned, too much in shock to move or speak. Then somebody ushered us into a waiting room. They said the surgery could last five to ten hours depending on complications. This was the marathon we'd been in training for, the race we never wanted to enter.

Everybody had cell phones, which you are not allowed to use in the hospital. They went outside and started making calls: to Lauren in California and to the airlines to confirm her emergency flight, to the G'parents and Uncle Sam to get them here safely as soon as possible. There was a flurry of activity around me but I was too burned out to move. I'd spent way too many hours trying to "sleep" in these uncomfortable chairs. Other families started to arrive. They looked like experienced waiting room occupants as well. They too settled in for a long haul. Somebody headed to the cafeteria for coffee and lousy food. We made small talk. Uncle Sam ordered a truckload of Chinese food to be delivered to the waiting room.

Hours went by, stilted conversation, meaningless chatter. What was it like for Mom, I wondered? Was surgery going okay? Did the heart fit? Was it right for her?

When I couldn't stand it anymore, I decided to go for a walk. The October morning was crisp and cool. The sun was shining and there was a slight breeze. It felt better to be outside, away from the hospital. I headed across the George Washington Bridge, walking at a fast clip. The leaves on the cliffs were just starting to turn colors. The huge flag waved lazily. Armed and uniformed military personnel scrutinized bridge traffic, a grim reminder of the recent 9/11 tragedies.

When I returned to the waiting room five hours had passed. And then Dr. Deng strode purposefully into the waiting room and headed directly for Dad. We held our breaths collectively and didn't resume breathing until he was finished. Mom was fine, the heart was perfect, everything went well, she would be moved shortly to the Transplant ICU, she would remain unconscious for at least twelve hours, she would be on a breathing machine, she would have lots of IV bottles and several chest tubes, but she was okay.

Dr. Deng took time to tell us that the next forty-eight hours were critical, that she would have the best of care. He encouraged us to talk to her, as he was certain that she could hear us. Exhale. Collective tears and expressions of gratitude to Dr. Deng, for his kindness and obvious caring, not just today, especially today, but for everything, for every time. He made sure we understood how hard this was going to be for Mom moving forward. We knew he would be there to help her through.

Throughout the day for brief intervals we were allowed to visit her. She was in a room just big enough for all of the equipment. Her nurse sat at her bedside and never left the room, calling out on the intercom system for supplies and medications. The other nurses brought them to her. She never left. She was a small woman, with a British accent and gray tight curly hair and glasses. She was calm, kind, confident, caring, comfortable and professional. She obviously knew what she was doing. She was worried about all of us. We must have looked a little ragged personally, beaten up emotionally. We had the sense that she had been through this before. We just felt better knowing she was with Mom.

At some point that evening I left the hospital to drive to JFK airport to pick up Lauren. What a relief it was to lay eyes upon my sister. Throughout the ordeal she has been the only person who made me feel remotely better about the bizarre and brutal routine our lives had become. It wasn't anything she said or did but I just didn't feel so alone when she was around.

When I reached JFK I had gotten two hours sleep the night before and had been up for twenty hours or so. I remember seeing how tired Lauren looked as I first glimpsed her at the terminal. It dawned on me that she had easily had as rough a day as I had, with the early morning phone call, subsequent scramble to line up a last minute cross-country flight and the trip itself. She looked pale, bedraggled and excited. Was Mom okay? Is she going to be okay?

When we arrived back at the hospital it was close to midnight, and the G'parents, Aunt Mare and Uncle Sam had gone home. Mom woke up when Lauren and I walked into the room.

I had seen Mom briefly in recovery just before I left for the airport. There was so much pressure wrap, gauze, tubing and respiration equipment wrapped around her upper torso that she looked as though she had on football shoulder pads under a white jersey. There was a breathing tube in her mouth that was taped in place that really bothered me. It just looked so alien and uncomfortable. Her eyes were still half closed and I gathered that she was still feeling the effects of the anesthesia. I gripped her hand but could not tell definitively if she knew I was there.

When I re-entered the room with Lauren later that night, her eyes opened a little wider and the look of recognition and happiness was unmistakable. She couldn't talk but she gripped our hands with surprising strength while we talked to her. The feeling in the room was electric. We were exhausted, elated, upset by how life-&-death serious Mom's situation had become and cautiously optimistic that a turn of events so positive, hopeful and utterly pivotal had occurred. After weeks of slow decline this was the event that could change everything dramatically for the better.

The nurses kept the visit short and we were ushered out of the room. In the hallway a feeling of relief hit me. With the slight release in tension I suddenly felt so tired that I couldn't see straight. Lauren and Dad drove east together to my folks' place in Huntington. I drove back over the GW Bridge to New Jersey and called my friend Lauren Elizabeth (now my wife) and asked to sleep on her couch in Gladstone rather than drive all the way to the G'parents' house. After spending so many nights over the previous weeks sleeping alone in random places (motels, the hospital waiting room, my car, etc.) it was a nice feeling to have someone expecting me and excited to see me. She waited up and we spent a few minutes talking before I passed out in a fitful sleep.

– *Brad Moose*
Summer 2004

♥

"When I returned to the waiting room five hours had passed.
And then Dr. Deng strode purposefully into the waiting room and headed
directly for Dad. We held our breaths collectively and didn't resume
breathing until he was finished. Mom was fine, the heart was perfect, every-
thing went well, she would be moved shortly to the Transplant
ICU, she would remain unconscious for at least twelve hours, she would
be on a breathing machine, she would have lots of IV bottles and
several chest tubes, but she was okay.

———————————————

"But those who wait on the Lord shall renew their strength;
they shall mount up with wings like eagles, they shall run and not be weary,
they shall walk and not faint." – Isaiah 40:31

— ♥ —

14   THE STRENGTHENED HEART

Wednesday, October 3, 2001 –

Two days post-transplant

After two days in the Transplant Intensive Care, I was moved to a critical care step-down unit with four beds. Two of my roommates were young men, ages 18 and 27. I was old enough to be their mother. Both had been transplanted the same weekend that I was. My heart went out to them. My third roommate was a man about my own age or a little younger. He had had bypass surgery for coronary vessel disease. I remember feeling as though we were all emerging from a fog. Things seemed more real and more normal, as in the aftermath of a hurricane. We had survived. We were all in pretty tough shape to be sure, we four roommates, but we were alive both individually and collectively. We seemed to draw on each other's strength and share in each other's pain.

We all had multiple chest tubes for drainage, as well as big chest incisions. We were expected to use our spirometers to aerate our lungs and to cough hourly to force secretions out of our lungs. Obviously, coughing was very painful. NYPH/C provided stuffed Teddy bears with NYPH/C T-shirts to hold tightly to our chests to minimize the discomfort. I had been in the middle of an asthma exacerbation immediately prior to and during my surgery. I wheezed when I coughed and sometimes couldn't readily stop coughing due to the irritation in my lungs.

On my first day in this unit, one of my coughs dislodged a chest tube and all of a sudden I was in extreme pain. We were expected to breathe deeply into the spirometer to reach a volume of 1200cc. We came close but had to struggle to do so. Following that painful cough, I could only achieve a volume of 250cc. I knew that if I couldn't expand my lungs I was at risk of developing pneumonia – a condition that would be fatal to me given my debilitated condition.

The other medical dilemma concerned the amount of drainage that was flowing from the pleural space in my chest. Chest tubes cannot be removed until drainage ceases, for fear it will accumulate and cause a pneumothorax, or collapsed lung. And I still needed the tubes for drainage.

Over the course of the next seemingly interminable hours I sat on the side of my bed, unable to breathe any more than 200cc into my lungs, and still in extreme pain. My nurse periodically offered pain medication. On several occasions she notified one of the interns or residents on call – who of course would not dare to interfere with the case of a fresh transplant. Only the transplant surgeon himself could make decisions about my care, and he was in surgery. I sat on the side of my bed rolling and unrolling a roll of tape, crying. My roommates murmured words of support and encouragement. They didn't get any rest either, out of concern for me.

At last, my transplant surgeon Dr. Naka got out of surgery and came to my bedside. Despite the risk of pneumonthorax he ordered that the chest tube be removed. The pain immediately disappeared. My lungs remained fully expanded without the tubes. One more hurdle cleared.

At this point in the recovery process, day two post-transplant, my roommates and I were expected to get out of bed and begin to walk. My legs were like tree trunks, filled with fluid all the way up to my groin. They seemed to weigh one hundred pounds apiece – the yield of copious intravenous fluids given during surgery and generally taking several days to be excreted from the body. I couldn't walk by myself because I had no idea what my legs were going to do, so unaccustomed was I to their bulk and their weight. The physicians ordered high doses of Lasix, a powerful diuretic, to expedite the process. I lost seventeen pounds in one day.

Jim and Lauren assisted me in our short walks around the unit. The enormity of the surgery wasn't the issue; rather I was so weak from the long siege of being critically ill. At the same time I was exhilarated. I wasn't short of breath. My nail beds were pink. When the phlebotomist drew my blood, I marveled at the rich, red color. The defibrillator device that had been in my heart was gone and I was in a normal, fast rhythm. During surgery, the vagus nerve, a major cranial nerve responsible for slowing down heart rate, is cut so the transplanted heart has a resting pulse of about 100 beats per minute – 40 beats per minute more than previously. It takes some getting used to. You have to start out slow, give your heart a chance to catch up to the demand and then cool down when you are done, giving your heart a chance to slow down again.

As we collectively began to heal, I got to know my three roommates. The young man we called the "ambassador" was our leader. He was determined to get back home to his wife and young child. He walked around our room and out to the unit to encourage the other patients who were still waiting for their hearts. One woman had been on the unit for seven months waiting for her heart. Others had waited varying lengths of time for theirs. We knew, with sadness, that some of these people might not survive the long wait.

As it happened, all of the heart patients seemed to congregate in our room. The youngest of us was a Latin American teenager. His parents did not speak English and both had to work long hours, so they weren't there very much. He had been sick a long time. His recovery was not progressing as well as ours were. He was discouraged. He touched our hearts. We all reached out to him. Our "ambassador" figured out how to get more and better food out of the kitchen and ordered extra for him. His wife even bought this teenager a pair of sneakers, which the staff required us to walk in instead of slippers lest we fall. The staff and the patients did all that they could to encourage him.

One of the waiting heart patients brought in crayons and Halloween character worksheets, purple-ink mimeographs that I can still see in my mind, for all of us to color. It was a mindless but life-affirming activity. We could now all do this small thing. It was a huge blessing. We did it together, just as we had in Kindergarten. One of the nurses spent all her free time with that thoughtful young man, in her quiet way encouraging him to keep fighting. Though it felt like the aftermath of a hurricane, this stage of recovery is in fact the eye of the storm. There is still a long way to go. The kindly nurse hung our completed pictures around the nurses' station.

Thursday, October 4 –
Three days post-transplant

My daughter called in the morning to say that our cat, Mitten, had been put to sleep by the veterinarian. She was nineteen years old and had gone into kidney failure. Lauren has a real affinity for cats and was shocked and distressed when she arrived from California, on the evening of the transplant, to find Mittie so sick. She said that Jim and Brad were in such terrible shape themselves, not having slept or eaten much for close to two months, that they didn't notice that Mittie was sick. Before coming to the hospital that morning, Lauren and Brad drove Mitten to our veterinarian. I cried and cried and cried when I heard. My roommates felt terrible for my loss and I felt terrible about disturbing them, but I couldn't seem to help myself. I pulled the curtain closed and I cried because I knew I would never see Mittie again. I cried because there was yet another thing to suffer about. I cried just because I think I needed to. One of my former pastors called and offered to pray with me. I asked him to pray for my kitty. I can picture her now, purring softly in heaven.

Friday, October 5 –
Four days post-transplant

Today – four days post-transplant – we were moved out of the step-down unit onto the regular hospital floor. We were all placed in rooms on 7 Hudson North, so were still near each other. The young men asked for a room together. I got a private room overlooking the Hudson River. For the first time in months it was quiet, the only sound the ringing telephone – finally, communication with the outside world! I relished the normalcy.

Our fourth roommate was just across the hall. On our exercise forays we always sought each other out, exchanging cards, specific colors of crayons and information. Now the goal was to get home. But not everything was going well. The "ambassador" was running a fever. The young man needed more chemotherapy. The fourth roommate was still having considerable pain.

We were all assigned to a wonderful nurse, Paquita, who cajoled us, teased us, tested us and generally helped us to feel normal again. Her smile worked its wonders on us. She tried to prepare us for going home. She was determined that we would learn our medications, many in number, spread out throughout our day and varied in function – very confusing, even for a nurse like me. She would deliver our meds and tell us to check them and take them only if we were sure they were correct. When she saw us coming to find her, she knew we had gotten it right; we had picked up her deliberate error. When our young friend had to have chemotherapy, he withdrew and became very depressed. Paquita stayed close to his side, performing all of her other duties, but hovering near him, keeping an eagle eye. She holds a special place in my heart.

Saturday-Wednesday, October 6-10

Five days post-transplant, and beyond . . .

I asked Jim to bring in my Bible. For the first time, I was strong enough to hold it in my hands. I turned to the book of Philippians, a favorite of mine. My attention span was short from both the medications and the lengthy illness. I embraced this short book, reading it over and over trying hard to remember the wisdom in its passages. It brought me great comfort.

One benefit of the private room was that Jim and I could be alone for the first time in months. He had been afraid to touch me since that terrible night in the Emergency Room when I was on fire, and since then because I was so fragile. But now, as I regained some of my strength, all I wanted was for him to hold me. In the silence of the darkened room, we watched the star-filled night and moonlight on the Hudson River. He said I was beautiful, which was of course not true. What he meant was that it was beautiful that I was alive.

One of the first things I noticed in my new room was a wonderful little sign on the wall, strategically placed at eye level when I was sitting up in bed. It said, "Dried fruits and nuts delivered in the afternoon daily." I couldn't believe my good fortune. Finally, something I could eat that was tasty, nutritious and filling. I was still starving.

The first day when the delivery didn't happen, I thought it was because I had missed the volunteer because I was out walking. The second and third days I made a point of staying in my room, doing my exercises at bedside. By the fourth day, I began to realize it wasn't going to happen. Rather than ask Jim for one more thing, I adjusted my expectations to fit the situation. I just couldn't handle another gastronomic disappointment. As it turned out I couldn't have eaten them anyway – too much potassium! I can laugh about this today. . . .

Friday, October 12

Discharge day! I was filled with anticipation and fear. I was afraid to leave and terrified to stay. The fact that Dr. Deng would be my post-transplant physician gave me the courage to leave. I knew he would be available when I needed him, this extraordinary man. The transplant team has a well-designed system whereby a patient can get in touch with a transplant physician 24/7. Built into the discharge plan were detailed instructions on how to call, when to call, what to report and when to come back in for clinic appointments; I was scheduled to return in three days for a cardiac biopsy. The nurses hand you a bag filled with an array of medications, and must be confident that thanks to your post-transplant training you know exactly what they are and exactly how and when to take them, before they will let you go home. Despite all of their wonderful education, it was a huge emotional hurdle for me to leave their care.

I left the hospital and Jim drove me to my parents' home in northern New Jersey, where I would stay until I was well enough to climb the stairs in our Long Island house.

"We were all assigned to a wonderful nurse, Paquita, who cajoled us,
teased us, tested us and generally helped us to feel normal again. Her smile
worked its wonders on us. She tried to prepare us for going home.. . ."

_____

"I can do all things through Christ
who strengthens me." – Philippians 4:13

———— 💜 ————

15 LETTER TO MY PARENTS

October 1

Dear Mom and Dad,

I can't imagine what it is like to lose a child, but I know you came awfully close to finding out. I'm so sorry I put you through so much pain, and so grateful that you took me home to recover until I was well enough to go home to Long Island. The responsibility for my care must have frightened you, yet you never appeared overwhelmed. How courageous you were to accept me.

Dad, you performed admirably well as my "Head Nurse," acting as a buffer between me and the outside world that could provide risk or simply tire me. Mom, your attention to my dietary and spiritual needs was so much appreciated. I know neither of you believes that my thanks are necessary, but for my sake, please let me put pen to my thoughts and my thanks.

I remember, as Jim and I waited for the hospital valet service to bring the car up from the parking lot, the breeze against my cheek. There was a time when I thought I might never feel that feeling again. Summer had changed to autumn. The day had shortened to late afternoon. I had lost a whole season of my life.

Jim strapped me into the seatbelt with my NYPH/C Teddy bear gripped tightly to my chest. I was anxious to leave, but scared to death to drive away from the kindly and capable medical professionals I had grown to depend on. In the car, I was finally alone with Jim after two long months.

We left the City just ahead of rush hour. I remember arriving at your house on the hill right on the heels of a FedEx truck. The uniformed man in shorts and shirtsleeves jumped out of his truck and dashed toward the door. Just as he reached the first step, you opened the door and your two sweet dogs lunged forward, barking excitedly at my arrival. The poor FedEx man bolted back into his truck, oblivious to the significance of my arrival, understandably fearful for his own safety. He gingerly passed the package out of a crack in the window and left. We all started to laugh, inappropriate though it may have been.

Our laughter progressed to hysterical tears as the dogs played at my feet, vying for my attention. The tension of the moment faded away. I was safely home with you.

You had purchased a bed for me, and set up a room for me in your first-floor study because I couldn't manage the stairs to reach the second floor. Sorry to displace you, Dad. For the next seven weeks this was my home and I was your problem. Jim went back to work and came out on weekends.

How intrusive it must have been to have so many strangers in and out of your house in those ensuing weeks. Medical professionals came almost daily to draw blood, administer chemotherapy, monitor my progress and direct my physical therapy program. I loved walking in your beautiful yard, first once around the pool and then around and around, reaching up to ring the wind chimes with each lap, increasing the number daily as my strength improved. Do you remember the day the big black bear walked out of the woods nearby and right up the driveway, minutes after I had come in from doing my laps? We just missed each other – bears are commonplace in these woods and I was just a visitor. What a sight!

I know I distressed you by being so emotional. When the nurse practitioner called and said I had to be readmitted for severe rejection, I fell apart. I'd been out of the hospital for only three days, and now I had to go back in. I was afraid I would never come out again; but I did. I remember Rev. Luthman saying, "There must be some more work that God needs you to do there."

I know I cried a lot during those seven weeks – tears of joy, tears of grief, tears of weariness. I grieved for the parents who gave me their son's heart. I was spent, physically and emotionally, and with chemotherapy and steroids and sleep interrupted to receive them, I was all over the map. In retrospect, I think I was in shock. So much had happened so fast, and I never saw it coming. No excuses, however – I know it must have been hard for you to see me that way. But there was nowhere else I could have gone, and there was nowhere else I wanted to be.

Mom, thanks for doing all the little Mom things that you do best: helping me with my bath, making my meat well done and unsalted and peeling my fruit to make it safely germ-free for me to eat. Thanks too for arranging for me to be anointed with oil, and to have communion at home. Thanks for all the little things you did for my comfort and for my soul. Dad, thanks for taking me out for rides in the car, for fixing my glasses and staying up late with me to watch the Yankees, for all your acts of kindness and care. It was a very special time.

Do you remember the night of the meteor shower? Jim and I got up at 2 a.m. to watch the stars race across the sky. We stood there in the dark and held each other, marveling at the display of God's creation.

I know you were reluctant to see me go, that you didn't think I was ready to go home. My desire to be with Jim was not a desire to leave you but rather a blessed wish to be reunited with my husband, to return to my life on Long Island at last.

I thank God for you, for your wonderful gifts of healing. I will always remember this time when we struggled together to get back my health. I Love You With All My (New) Heart.

– Your Daughter, Candace
Fall 2004

"I loved walking in your beautiful yard, first once around the pool and then around and around, reaching up to ring the wind chimes with each lap, increasing the number daily as my strength improved. . . ."

_____

*"To everything there is a season, a time for every purpose under heaven:
a time to heal, a time to build up, a time to laugh and a time to dance,
a time to embrace, a time of peace."* – Ecclesiastes 3:1, 3, 4, 5, 8

16 EMBRACING MY NEW HEART

October-November 2001 and Beyond

I learned so many new things in my weeks of hospital time and first steps of recovery at my parents' house. The complexities of this diagnosis, transplant surgery and recovery seemed sensible yet infinite, oftentimes overwhelming. One step I had yet to make was to write the letter of gratefulness to my donor family, which I felt was part of the process of daring to embrace my new heart as my own.

There are only two pieces of information that the medical staff is allowed to give you after a transplant, and they are the sex and age of the organ donor. When they woke me up to tell me my new heart was on the way and surgery was scheduled for the morning, I knew in my heart, as I have mentioned, that it was a child, a teenager. My grief for the family of that child was overwhelming – I couldn't get my arms around the fact that a young life had had to end in order for a fifty-year-old woman to live. Had I been doing the choosing, I would have given my life for that child. But I am not in charge, so grief and gratefulness were mixed profoundly in my mind. I knew I would try to tell this to my donor family.

Through the Transplant Clinic at NewYork-Presbyterian, and in conjunction with the New York Organ Donor Network, there is as noted a mechanism whereby a transplant recipient can write a thank-you letter to a donor family. The letter is screened by three independent reviewers to make sure all pertinent geographical and personal information that could link the two parties is not present, so that confidentiality is maintained.

I did write several weeks after surgery. It was the hardest task I have ever undertaken. How exactly do you say thank-you for such a gift? What can you say? I wrote that I would try to live my life to be worthy of such a gift. I have not received a response and I don't expect one, knowing that this family must be consumed by grief. But someday perhaps I will hear from them. Later I did write again. If both the donor family and the recipient choose to have their identities revealed to the other, the NYODN will bring them together – otherwise both parties remain anonymous. It is, appropriately, a very individual decision.

I've met a number of donor moms and dads in my recovery. Their grief is palpable. I tell them who I am, what happened to me and how much I appreciate their courage and their generosity. I try to tell them in person because I cannot do so to the family that gave so generously to me. Some parents have revealed that they did not receive letters of thanks from their recipients. I offer the possible explanation that the patient may have been too ill to write, knowing how unwell I was for months afterward.

The first six months following any transplant, I have learned, are a critical time. Recovery is a full-time job, from tracking medications, to preparing special foods, to physical therapy, to rest, to doing the things that heal your heart and nourish your soul. Lots of things go wrong. The medications are harsh, causing side effects. Lab values fluctuate. Low white cell counts leave recipients at risk for infections, isolating them from the outside world. Low red cell counts and immunosuppressive drugs cause fatigue, limiting activity. Chemotherapy and Prednisone cause insomnia and other drugs cause many more unfamiliar and uncomfortable side effects. It's a scary time. Clinic visits back to the doctor are frequent; initially weekly, then biweekly, then monthly. Traveling to the City for these visits is hard, disruptive to the recovery routine and tiring. Tests are invasive, exhausting and anxiety provoking.

Heart transplant patients have cardiac biopsies regularly to test for rejection. In my case, the physicians are also testing for the return of the disease that destroyed my first heart, giant cell myocarditis. Then there are the psychological issues of recovery. Initially most of us ask, What happened to me and why?

The next level of questions has to do with recovery. Why, if I am doing everything the doctors said, am I not better? Why do things keep going wrong? Will I ever be "better"? At the deepest level, somewhere within the course of the illness or recovery, the questions regarding our ultimate mortality surface. Does this new heart work? How long will it work? Am I prepared to die? Most of us have come very close to doing just that.

And finally, when we do get well, we attempt to answer questions about the future. Why did I live? What am I supposed to do with this second chance? What is the purpose not just of my life but of existence overall? Some of us have sought counseling in an attempt to deal with the emotional stress of our traumatic illness.

As I progressed in my own recovery over the course of the next year, I reached a point where I wanted to know more. My doctor informed me that my donor had in fact been seventeen years old. This new information was a validation of what I already knew deep inside. It caused another wave of grief to flood over me. For months afterward, I thought of that child, of my own children at age seventeen and of my friend's daughter who had died at age twenty-one of leukemia, and another friend's son who died at age thirteen from another form of cancer. They say that there is no grief more profound than that of parents whose child precedes them in death. Many times throughout my illness I have been grateful that it happened to me and not to my children. There is something intrinsically wrong with the illness and death of children. It is out of order. It is unfair. It seems, somehow, a more profound tragedy than the death of someone older.

Almost two years before learning more, I had also sensed this was the heart of a boy. My thoughts never entertained the possibility that the donor was a girl; I don't know why. I dreamed that he was a popular high school boy who played sports, probably golf, tennis and possibly a running position on the football team. He was also a leader, a class officer or student government officer. In my dreams I not only pictured him physically, as obviously we were the same height and weight, but I felt as though I knew him personally. Though I couldn't see his face, I knew his heart. I found myself always thinking about this young man. I welcomed him like a friend. He is with me everywhere, in my waking and in my dreams. In my prayers today I thank not only his family for this gift, but also him as well – embracing all the aspects of his life – for giving me a second chance at mine.

People have asked me whether I noticed anything different about having someone else's heart beat in my chest. Did I suddenly crave beer and pizza? Did I discover that I liked murder mysteries, which I previously hated? No, not beer and pizza and mystery stories. But it's not a frivolous question, as I have learned.

My friend Kathleen drove me to a driving range many times that first summer after the transplant, when my chest had healed sufficiently for this type of exercise. From the very first stroke, after at least three or four years of not having picked up a club, my swing was close to perfect. Ball after ball flew straight as an arrow, 100-150 yards out. I was surprised and confused as well as a little embarrassed by this newfound talent. While my friend struggled to find her groove, I continued this previously elusive trend.

Finally, Kathleen voiced her frustration at her own lack of performance and my enhanced performance and basically said, "What gives?" Sheepishly, I answered that the only thing I could think of is that with the gift of the new heart, I was also given my donor's golf skills. It was an epiphany of sorts, as I was uncertain whether I could trust what I was daring to say. Was it possible to receive other things from a donor than just the organ? Was I imagining all of this? I have learned so much since that first questioning time. Oftentimes, other transplant recipients have stated, skills and cravings do appear to come with a transplanted organ. Current research is discovering why this may be.

It was on a later visit to the City to see Dr. Deng, that I asked him the sex of my donor and he confirmed it was a boy. "I knew it!" I exclaimed. He said that changing a heart was not at all the same thing as changing an engine in a car. We as human beings are so much more complex than inanimate objects. That there are many unexplained or imperceptible phenomena in an organ transplant. He asked if I thought of this person as a mother would think of a child. I said, no, that I embraced this teenager as a friend. Every time I think of him, I smile. I think of him with love, respect and wonder.

Dr. Deng said that how positively we think of the new organ, whether or not we accept someone else's organ in our body, may affect our future health. He said that some patients fight their new organs; they cannot accept the organ as their own, but view it as an adversary. He was suggesting that sometimes how we view the foreign organ on an intellectual level might well influence how our body accepts or rejects the organ on a tissue level.

Rejection, the NYPH/C manual explains, is an ongoing concern throughout the life of a transplant patient. Rejection means that the immune system has recognized the foreign organ as an invader and as such mounts an attack to destroy the invader. To minimize the chances of transplant rejection, physicians seek to match donor organs that share as many biochemical properties as possible with the transplant recipient's. Even so, all transplant recipients must take immunosuppressive drugs for the rest of their lives. The doctors attempt to control the rejection of the organ by balancing the biopsy results against the toxic side effects of the drugs.

Uncontrolled or inadequately treated rejection can lead to organ failure.

At the same time, by definition, the drugs are suppressing the recipient's immune system and therefore compromising the body's ability to fight off infection of all types. A transplant person must always be vigilant about exposure to infectious diseases. I avoid public places in flu season. If my white blood cell counts are below the normal limits, a side effect of the combinations of drugs I take, I either stay home or wear a mask if I have to go out in public. I scope out every public situation to ascertain whether anyone is visibly ill. I quietly leave if I discover people coughing or if I see an unusual rash.

Frequent hand washing is one of the best defenses against communicable disease. I wash all raw fruits and vegetables. I peel everything that can be peeled. All meat and seafood has to be cooked well done. I take antibiotics prior to dental work. For the first year following the transplant I didn't clean my house, garden, go near a construction site, have cut flowers in my house, handle raw meat or go near young children. I couldn't even touch my beloved dog Ruffie. My counts are up now, so some of these restrictions have lifted – but I remain vigilant.

Probably most importantly for me, there will be no future travel to third world countries, so Africa is out. I cannot ever receive the vaccines required for travel, nor could I be that far away from expert medical care anyway. The whole experience comes full circle. Gratefully I am well again. I like to say, "New and improved." Some strides have been made in fighting the AIDS pandemic in Africa, but not enough. I am sad that I cannot directly participate in this world-important fight. But I am profoundly thankful for my gift of life, and determined to use it for good purpose.

"But to you who fear My name the Sun of Righteousness
shall arise with healing in His wings." – Malachi 4:2

———— ❦ ————

17   THE HEALING HEART

As I look back on my recovery since the transplant, I recall my messages of
love received and love reciprocated, and the ups and downs of the difficult recovery. E-mails from these months are for me a story in themselves. I include some
here – messages to family, friends and colleagues – that are unwitting foreshad-
owings and highlights of the journey that took us all by surprise. I include some
e-mails to Dr. Deng as well.

□

Pre-transplant –
July 9, 2001
Dear Dee:
(Church friend, California)
    I've been asked to go to Malawi with a group called Save the Children.
Through the Presbyterian Church USA, I have engaged our church in collecting
sheets for hospitals in Malawi and the Democratic Republic of the Congo. I've
made myself available to the PC United Nations office. I'm always most comfort-
able operating within a church organization, so I have to carefully consider
whether or not to accept this opportunity. Please pray for me.

□

August 14

Dear Dee:

Other news: I have made the decision to go to Africa with Save the Children to visit AIDS impact areas in Malawi at the end of September and, on a lighter note, I am taking rowing lessons. First, Africa. I will be working with the Presbyterian Church United Nations office on AIDS in Africa starting in September. I called to volunteer and they took me up on my offer. When the trip came up with the Save the Children folks, they asked and I said yes. I am really scared to death, but going anyway because I feel that this is what I have been called to do in my retirement (AIDS in Africa). Re: rowing, it is great fun. I wanted to see Long Island from the water. The whole experience is exhilarating. We row in the evening when the sun is setting. Exotic birds stand in the salt marshes as we row past. I love it.

☐

Post-Transplant –
November 26, 2001

Dearest Linda:
(Church friend, California)

Your prayers and those of many others, including mine, have been answered by a gracious and loving God. I arrived home on Long Island Friday after a three-month absence, which included 53 days in the hospital and seven weeks of recuperation at my parents' home in New Jersey. I had to be able to walk up a flight of stairs before I could come home. I have a new heart!

Recovery is slower than I expected. They said the first year would be hell. But I am grateful for every day. Please keep praying for me, dear friend, I know God hears. Now that I am home, we can e-mail. Thanks sooo much for your cards. They meant so much to me in my darkest hours.

☐

November 30

Dearest Ro:

(Former professional colleague)

I came home to Jim on Long Island one week ago today after a three-month absence. It's been quite an experience, but I am improving daily. The chemo takes a lot out of me and the immunosuppressant meds have unpleasant side effects. I finished five treatments of one kind and have the sixth treatment to go of the second kind, ending just before Christmas. If the pathology reports continue to be negative for giant cell in the new heart, I won't need any more. That is our prayer. I've been given a second chance to live! I thank God every day for today.

☐

December 1

Dear Linda:

Third world countries are out forever. In fact, I can only vacation to places in the U.S. and the world that have heart transplant centers nearby — which, by the way, includes Los Angeles. I walk for 30 minutes every day and do physical therapy at home. I am feeling better every day.

☐

December 6

Dearest Don and Ann:

(Church friends, California)

Since my return to Long Island last week, I have been reading all of the cards and letters that were sent to me during my hospitalization. Jim saved them for me. I'm about 1/2 of the way through. Notice I did not say re-reading, as so many I do not remember at all. Maybe some days I was too sick for Jim to read them to me. The curiosity is that I thought I was lucid the whole time.

Anyway, my point is that I am humbled and deeply touched by your frequent and faithful expressions of love over the past months. I had you in my heart. I knew you were next to me every minute. I just did not know how often you wrote to tell me. . . .

□

December 11

Dear Diane:

(Neighborhood friend, California)

Had a little scare that ended up being nothing. New York called on Friday to say that I had a spot on my lung, which showed up on the chest x-ray. I went in yesterday for a CAT scan and it turned out to be negative. Thank you, God. Feeling great!

Just finished re-reading all my wonderful cards. The pictures of us at the Yankee game and in New York are wonderful. Playing the piano almost every day and listening to Christmas carols. I love Christmas! Lauren comes in next week and I have my last chemo (I hope) next Wednesday. They sent my (old) heart and all of my (new) heart biopsies off to Mayo Clinic for a second opinion. All of New York's biopsies have been negative for giant cell. Let's hope Mayo reads them the same. My love to everyone. Love you all dearly!

□

December 12

Dear Moose family:

(Jim's extended family)

After six weeks with my parents in New Jersey, I'm home on Long Island with Jim after a three-month absence. It's taken a little time to get organized and to feel well enough to get back on e-mail, but here I am — with a new heart. I am doing well; a little better every day. . . . I walk 30-45 minutes a day and have folks who come into our home to do physical therapy, blood work and chemo. I am an eating machine. My resting heart rate in the new heart is almost twice what it was in my old heart, so consequently, my metabolism is turned up. I eat six small meals a day. Believe or not, my days are full. Getting healthy is a full time job.

The doctors told me that my new heart was "beautiful." I didn't ask for any more details. Though I was elated to know that I finally had a chance to live, I felt such grief for the family of the donor who made such a courageous decision at what had to be the most tragic time of their lives. Please remember them in your prayers.

I would be remiss if I did not tell you that there were many blessings in the midst of the suffering. Exceedingly competent medical professionals and support staff who cared for me. Doctors and nurses who prayed with me and for me. A heart that was a perfect match that became available in less than two days when I was failing rapidly. It had to match by blood type, body height and weight. I'd lost so much weight since my admission that for me to be exactly the weight I needed to be a perfect match was nothing short of a miracle. And now I am home. I love being back in my own house, in my own bed, with my husband. I love the quiet, after months of bells, whistles and alarms. I love my piano. I play hymns and sing for my own enjoyment. Most of all, I love the great Healer/Physician who gave me a second chance. I find myself smiling all the time. There is such joy in my heart.

□

December 13

Dear Linda:

I'm not doing Christmas this year in the secular sense. I am simply not well enough and not allowed to be out in public due to my immunosuppression. Our holiday will be simply what I believe it was always intended to be, and that is celebration of the birth of the Christ child with loved ones; no gifts, no rushing around, no hoopla – just family. . . .

□

December 19

Dear Sue, Doug, Gene and Linda:
(Family)

I can't begin to tell you how much your cards and prayers meant to me. Since I'm not allowed out in public because of the immunosuppression, I have been baking my Christmas presents this year. I love tinkering in the kitchen. When we were first married and had no money, I would bake Christmas presents for everybody. Thirty years later, I'm doing it again. Though for a different reason, I'm enjoying every minute of it!

□

December 19

Dear Dr. Deng:

I decided to take you up on your offer and contact you via e-mail with some questions. I hope this is okay. Regarding the low WBC count, is this something you were expecting at this point? I'm a little surprised, but I also have no experience in chemotherapy. How long will it take for the count to return to normal? Will we go ahead with the last Cytoxan treatment when it does?

I called your nurse practitioner today and left a message to tell her that I have been having some lightheadedness, primarily on changing position from lying down to standing, and less so from sitting to standing. It is one of the symptoms listed in the NYPH/C manual that should be reported to your doctor. Everything else is good: weight is stable, ankles are fine.

My physical therapy is going well. I'm getting stronger by the day. Should I be exercising with this low white cell count or should I be backing off a bit? I'd like to start running as soon as I am able. I have a great therapist.

I will see you next week on the 27th for my clinic visit and biopsy, unless I hear something different from you in the meantime. Wishing you and your family a blessed holiday. And, as always, thank you for your wonderful care.

☐

December 21

Dearest Sue:

I believe that if I believe I am going to get well I will. That is the essence of faith. This whole thing has been a very spiritual experience.

☐

December 22

Dearest Ro:

Thank you for all of your love and prayers. . . . I feel really good now, but keep hitting these bumps in the road that force me to remember that I am not yet well. God keeps telling me, "I'm in charge." I have a great physical therapist who pushes me. As I cannot get outside the house to go to a cardiac rehab facility, we will continue to train at home. Believe it or not I want to begin running. For the first time in my life, I'm light enough to run. Just waiting for the doctor's permission.

☐

December 28

Dear Dr. Deng:

Needless to say, I am delighted with the negative biopsy results and increasing WBC. Sue [Dr. Deng's nurse practitioner, the very best!] said to decrease the Prednisone to 7.5mg BID starting tonight per your written instructions in my chart. Are these too many changes for my bone marrow at one time?

The other thing that I am concerned about is the abnormal ECG, which notes a right ventricular conduction problem in V1. I took the ECG home by accident yesterday after clinic and faxed it over this morning for your review.

Sorry to bother you with these things. I don't want to leave things hanging over a holiday weekend. We're on our way to Mother's for dinner and an overnight. We will probably be back to pick up your return e-mail message, if you choose to leave one by tomorrow night. Have a blessed, healthy and happy New Year and thank you for your always prompt and caring responses to my e-mails.

☐

December 30

Dear Joy:

(Former professional colleague)

Congratulations on the birth of your new grandchild. Hope all is well for both Mom and baby. . . . As I am not allowed in public, i.e., shopping in the malls, I made all my Christmas presents. You know how I have always loved tinkering in the kitchen. I am thankful for my piano, which I have the chance to play for the first time in years. And, I am determined to finally learn Spanish (I'm afraid I wasn't a very attentive student in high school). I also decided to finally read the entire Bible, some-

thing I should have done years ago. As an aside, I am also reading Harry Potter. I wanted to know what all the hype was about. The books are just wonderful. Well-deserved hype. I'm walking again, 45 minutes a day. Hope to start running soon. They have transplant Olympics in June in Florida. Maybe not this year because of my immunosupression, but next year I'm considering competing in the over 50 egg toss!

□

December 31
Dearest Dee:

Your Christmas presents arrived on the afternoon of Christmas Eve. Your gifts were so much appreciated and arrived at a low moment. You lifted our spirits.

It's been a tough holiday. Not just the isolation now (low white cells again!), but also the isolation to come until my count recovers. The bone marrow just has to come back on its own. Needless to say January travel is cancelled – an activity that the doctors last month had encouraged us to begin planning. No church, no movies, no malls, no alcohol, no out to dinner, no grocery store even. Sounds like a real pity party, doesn't it? I've moved from the grief and fear to the anger stage of my dealing with this. I hope I don't stay here long, I don't like it. On a more positive note, I am REALLY enjoying Harry Potter. Send more Potter books please!

□

January 2, 2002

Dear Dee:

I love the words you choose, so à propos: "the tyranny of my medical condition." Some days it does feel like that. Other days I feel so good that I forget about it and just go on about my business, tinkering in the kitchen or cleaning a closet. You have been the best friend and the most supportive person anyone could ever have. I've leaned on you awfully hard. You've helped me to laugh at myself when other people have felt sorry for me. That scares me. I don't want to deal with the reality of this illness every minute of the day. My physical therapy guy is coming so I've got to run. White cell count today is 5.1, coming up! I thank God for you and Craig every day.

□

January 2

Dear Linda:

Happy New Year to you as well! I feel wonderful, but my blood work is lousy, though on the mend. Christmas was exceedingly quiet. One of the deacons from my new church delivered the Christmas Eve service on tape so I got out my hymnbook and Bible and sang and followed along with the service. That was wonderful, I felt connected. It has been so hard not being able to go to church, going on five months. I've hardly ever missed a Sunday in my life.

□

January 8

Dear Dee:

Thanks so much for the next Harry Potter book. They are so cute. Great news from New York yesterday . . . CAT scan was completely negative (can you believe it? suspected lung mass issue – all well!). . . . We took a lot of hits in December, and I know I didn't always handle them well. No matter how hard I tried, they seemed to come faster than I could deal with. January is already looking good. Lauren came out for three days and we had a wonderful time. Jim and Brad are both still tired, but the Christmas break certainly did help tremendously. So much to be thankful for.

□

January 14

Dear Dee:

I drove myself to the local clinical lab today to have my blood drawn. My first time driving since August. I was doing great until I missed a step coming out of the building. I stumbled, but didn't fall. Every new thing that I do causes a little bit of anxiety. Thankfully, neurologically I am improving so I feel I can drive, at least locally, though I really don't have any place to go. When my counts come up, Jim and I will be able to go to the movies, which I know he will enjoy. And I will be able to go to the grocery store during low traffic times; can't wait to do that. Then I can cook to my heart's content.

□

January 15

Dear Bill and Ellen:

(Former pastor and his wife, New Jersey)

I received your book on labyrinths via FedEx yesterday afternoon. Thank you so much for helping me through this time. I'm like a sponge right now. I'm trying to absorb everything I can so I can come to some understanding of what God wants me to take away from this experience. Regarding the book, I believe that meditation is not only spiritual; it's also physically very healthy.

Several years ago, Lauren and I had come across a canvas labyrinth at a church in San Francisco. We read about it, but didn't walk it. I read about a quarter of the book this morning (one of the blessings of this time of my life is that I can sit down and read a morning away if I feel like it). Fascinating stuff. There don't appear to be any labyrinths on Long Island, so I'm thinking that as soon as I get well, I might make a trip to Connecticut (where the author is from) or New York to walk one of these things.

□

January 15

Dear Steve and Sam:

(Friends, California)

I don't know where to begin. First, I want to thank you for all of your prayers and concern for me and for Jim over these past few months. Second, I want to tell you how wonderful I feel, so that you will not need to worry a moment longer than necessary. Since October 1st, we have a real good chance for an almost normal life. Without the gift from an anonymous family, we had no chance at all. We have been blessed, but we are fully cognizant of the fact that my gift of life came at a tremendous cost to someone else. It has been a very humbling experience. . . . We're coming to California as soon as I get clearance from the doctors. Right now my bone marrow isn't behaving so I am in isolation at home. Normally, transplant patients can return to work at six months, so I'm shooting for travel sometime late this spring.

□

January 17

Dear Dee:

Lab reports came back yesterday not as good as I expected. When Lauren visited two weeks ago I was almost in normal limits: 6.8. Then last week I dropped to 5.1 and this week I'm 4.1, so movies and the public in general continue to be not a possibility for me. Anyway, I feel wonderful, so that's that.

□

January 17

Dear Ro:

A friend sent me a card yesterday with an inscription written by Maya Angelou. It said that we can be changed by what happens to us, but we must refuse to be beaten by it. It goes on to say that we should be confident of two things: we are stronger than we think and we are never alone. Good stuff. I'm looking into participating in the Transplant Olympics in Florida in June. You do not compete against other athlete/transplant patients. Medals are awarded based on beating your own best times. Isn't that cute?

□

January 23

Dearest Pumpkin:

My biopsy results came back today 1A, which according to the book means no rejection. How it differs from O I don't know. Will find out tomorrow when Daddy and I talk to Dr. Deng. I don't know whether to be joyful or concerned that there is some rejection. We'll be off to New York at 5:45 a.m. Should be home around noon or 1 p.m. I will e-mail you then. Love you, my very special daughter, with all my heart.

□

January 24

Dear Lauren:

We just got back from the City. Daddy and I had a long talk with Dr. Deng. He's not concerned about rejection with the low white cell count, because he says the low count is what we want; however, it does leave me at risk for infection.

I told him I had started writing the book and that as research, for the first time I started looking up giant cell myocarditis on the internet. The information is not very encouraging. I asked him what my prognosis was. He answered with his gentle, encouraging smile that I should simply live every day as though it were my last. He suggested that Daddy do the same. There is no data available on long-term survival of giant cell folks who have had heart transplants.

He said people who have survived the kind of ordeal that I have are often changed by the experience. He said that I should do exactly what I want to do and not what other people want me to do. The problem is that what I want is for Daddy to retire and for us to live in a house between you and Brad so that I can be a grand-mother to both of your children. I have no desire to climb Mt. McKinley and trek the Appalachian Trail. I just want weddings and grandchildren and Dad. Pretty simple, don't you think?

□

January 25

Dearest Pumpkin:

Was having a great day. New York just called. WBC even lower, out of normal range. They're cutting four of my medications to non-therapeutic levels and upping the blood draws to twice a week. Their message: be careful, stay put. I can do that. I'm so busy with my Spanish tapes, piano practice, physical therapy, baking, Bible study and writing that I don't have time to feel bad.

☐

January 31

Dear Sunshine:

I've been in the kitchen this morning baking away, which I always love doing. Uncle Sam brought some bananas the other night when they came for dinner so I thought I'd make banana bread. Daddy bought me zucchini at the grocery store the other day which I now can't eat because my potassium is up, so I made zucchini bread. Time flies when I am having so much fun. Only one casualty, I burned myself on the oven rack. The visible tremors (common response to my meds) are mostly gone but I still spill everything, drop everything and bump into everything. I simply can't be trusted!

☐

February 7

Dear Lauren:

I'm trying hard not to panic. I just got a call from my GYN. I had a routine mammogram yesterday morning. And as you know I'm more susceptible to cancer of every kind, because of the immunosuppressive drugs. They want to take another set of films. They are not sure about the right breast. The soonest appointment I could get for a repeat test is Tuesday morning. So, another long weekend while we play this out. I think God has renamed me Job. I'll talk to you tonight.

February 11

Dear Williams Women:

Thank you so very much for the wonderful presents. What a marvelous surprise! You made my day. I felt as though it was my birthday. In college, we used to celebrate half-birthdays – any excuse to order a cake. I love the Fresh Produce dress. I promise to wear it for you when we come out in May, Lord willing. . . . You are right, Dee; I want to hang the dish on the wall. I'll have to send Jim to the hardware store to find the dish hangers. He's got the grocery store down pat. Now it's time to expand his horizons! . . . One of the wonderful books I am reading was written by a female physician turned counselor who advised one of her patients to record in a daily journal the answers to the following three questions: What surprised you today? What inspired you today? And what touched you today? You did all three of those things for me in one fell swoop. Thank you for keeping me in your care. I love you all. I'm off for blood work!

□

February 12

Dear Dr. Deng:

A couple of issues that I am not sure should wait until I see you next week given the lab results of today. I am having a little (what I perceive to be) liver fullness/tenderness since Saturday or Sunday. It is so hard to figure out what to eat with a K at 5.5. I'm losing weight (140 lbs). Feel a little more tired, but not bad.

□

February 14

Dear Doozie:

I just got home from New York. Had the cardiac biopsy and the whole deal. Had a great day seeing Dr. Deng and his staff. I'm really tired so am going to take a nap now. Call me tonight if you have a chance. Dr. Deng said that if today's cardiac biopsy was good and if next week's breast biopsy was good and if my WBC went up and my K (potassium) went down, we could still go to Florida on March 11th. I feel great and that counts for a lot. God bless you. Call me tonight?

□

February 15

Dear Kids:

I just got a call from New York regarding yesterday's results. The biopsy was negative (down from 1A), the white cell count was 3.1 (up from 2.5), the K was 3.8 (down from 5.5) and the cholesterol was 179 (down from 200). It doesn't get any better than this; except maybe the WBC could be a lot higher! A quadruple good whammy! Praise the Lord!!! I'm off to take my nap. Ruffie already scoped out his space. I love you both with all my heart.

□

February 15

Dearest Dee:

All good news from New York! The staff couldn't get over how good I look. I suspect they say that to all the patients. My friend from church who drove me in said I looked tons better than when she drove me in three weeks ago. It's hard to have an accurate perspective when you spend so much time alone. I don't even recognize the person in the mirror. Enough about me, except to say that I still need your prayers, and I know I have them.

February 19

Dear Michelle:

(Fellow heart transplant recipient)

It was such a nice surprise to run into you and your husband the other day in the clinic. So glad that you are finally home. You look wonderful. It was such a big step for me to come home. Part of me was afraid. Everything new throws me for a loop. I'd forgotten how much I love my own bed, not to mention having my husband within arm's reach. My puppy dog sleeps curled up at my feet. They both snore just a little. What wonderful sounds after all those bells and whistles. Please write or call if you feel like it, otherwise I'll just jot you off a note every now and then. Give my best regards to your Dad and your husband. God bless you and keep you.

□

February 22

Dear Lauren:

I hope you got some much-needed rest last night. We're so proud of how you did in the job interview. I told Dad what I could remember of your answers and he was impressed. I just got a call from Brad. He got an excellent performance rating and an 8% raise! What a kid! Given what he (and all of us) has been through these last six months, that kind of performance rating is pretty amazing. He said they weren't paying very close attention. . . . I got this far in the e-mail and Dr. Harris just called. The breast biopsy is negative. Praise the Lord! (I'm crying.) Some type of sclerosing something-or-other. Doozie I love you so much. I want to be your Mom for a long, long time. I can no longer see through my tears so I'm going to sign off. I love you. – Mom

□

"Behold, I stand at the door and knock.
If anyone hears My voice and opens the door, I will come in to him
and dine with him, and he with Me." – Revelation 3:20

———❤———

18 THE RESURRECTED HEART

Easter Sunday, March 31, 2002

My family and I attended Easter services at the church where my grandparents had belonged for fifty years. We were members of this church for the six years we lived in Sussex County, New Jersey.

What a glorious, glorious time we had that Easter morning. My grandfather, a Dutch immigrant, was a successful dairy farmer with a sixth grade education. At one point he owned the largest purebred registered Guernsey herd in the world. He purchased thirty farms in northern New Jersey that were roughly contiguous, amassing three thousand acres of property where he raised the cattle that produced the milk he sold.

The pasteurization plant was in North Haledon, where the milk was processed and then delivered to homes in Bergen and Passaic counties. My grandparents were great Christians. I grew up on their farm, along with my cousins and aunts and uncles. In many ways, it was an idyllic childhood. My cousins and I had the run of the farm: ponds to ice skate, hills to hike and sleigh ride, streams to fish, fields to ride, woods to explore, gardens to grow.

As a child, I would go to church with my grandparents whenever I could. The exterior of the First Presbyterian Church of Newton is made of blocks of granite.

The interior is elegantly appointed in dark wood and maroon carpeting. It is old and formal in both worship style and in architecture. It has a beautiful stained glass window of Jesus praying in the Garden of Gethsemane. The sound from the old pipe organ is enhanced by wonderful acoustics. I can't enter the church without thinking of my grandparents. They sat in exactly the same pew every Sunday. They were faithful, humble and generous people. I longed to live up to their expectations for me in my life.

Easter has never been more meaningful to me than it was this first spring after my new heart. I've tried unsuccessfully to understand the suffering of this past fall. It seemed to go on and on, one crisis after another, critical event followed by critical event. Why do we have to suffer? Do we have to be thrown to our knees in order to acknowledge God? Are we too busy with the business of life to be aware of God's presence in our lives?

The pastor's message this Easter morning was about the resurrection. About the fact that suffering is part of life. Whether it is illness or loss, poverty or danger, accident or injury, suffering is part of the human condition. Heaven is not here; our belief in the resurrection gives us the promise of eternal life. We will meet our loved ones again who have gone before us. We will look through the mirror of our misunderstandings and everything will become clear. Wrongs will be made right. Broken bodies and injured souls will be made whole. There will be no sorrow or pain. Our debts will be forgiven. We won't be limited by self-esteem, our race, our gender, our intelligence, our age, our health, and our finances or by anyone with power over us. There will be peace on earth and God will walk among us. This was our message on that comforting Easter Sunday.

"He makes me to lie down in green pastures;
He leads me beside the still waters, He restores my soul." – Psalm 23:2, 3

— ❤ —

19 THE HEALING HEART, PART 2

March 4, 2002

Dear Kathleen:

(Church friend, Long Island)

I was in church yesterday, in the balcony. We sat up there because I needed to stay away from children. We went early and picked a vacant spot. Just as the service was about to begin, three families walked in with five children and they sat behind, in front of and to the side of us. Oh well, I thought, God will take care of me. There was nary a cough or sneeze.

Had blood work drawn this morning; results will be back tomorrow afternoon. If all goes well we're scheduled to leave for Florida next Monday. Of course, I'm scared to death to fly – not terrorism, but infection. I want to get a new mask from the medical supply store – better filter. Anyway, I'm just wonderful today and so appreciative of your love and concern. I'm headed down to have lunch and then a nap! Just call me the princess and the pea.

□

March 4

Dearest Bill and Ellen:

Just checking in. A great day to be alive. It seems I've turned some kind of corner. After weeks of low blood counts, I'm noticing that as they come up, I feel better. . . .

□

March 8

Dearest Dee:

Spring is here! The sun is shining, the temperature is supposed to be low 60's and my spring bulbs are breaking through the ground. Better than that, I feel great. I ran my first fever since the transplant yesterday – a urinary tract infection that was quickly treated and resolved. Thank you God. Oh, and my counts are doing what they are supposed to do. . . . What I'm trying to get around to is an invitation – I think I'm ready for company. Can you guys come East in April? Lord willing, I think we're coming to you in May. We're leaving for Florida on Monday. . . . Jim is officially on vacation as of today and he is exhausted but exhilarated. I know I've said this to you before, but I think I am in better shape than all my family. I can't even imagine how difficult it must have been for them to be on the other side of the bed.

I saw an ad for Jet Blue on TV this morning: $109 each way from California to JFK. Please come. We miss you. I know it's not our prettiest season but there is plenty to do in New York. I probably won't sightsee with you, but I will have a wonderful dinner ready for you when you get home. There are all kinds of deals on theater tickets. Please, please come.

□

March 19

Dearest Joan:

We went to Florida on vacation with our children, had a wonderful time and my white cell count plummeted again. So I'm back home in isolation, but with an important difference – a tan!!!! I bought this high tech, ultra filter operating-room mask to wear in the airport and on the planes, so I felt pretty comfortable in public.

Did I tell you we would be celebrating our 30th wedding anniversary in June? We didn't want to wait to celebrate, hence the trip to Florida with our children last week. It was wonderful. I miss my daughter in Santa Barbara so very much, but we talk and e-mail every day. My son lives and works in New Jersey. Just to lay my eyes on them was a treat for my soul.

I'm off to New York on Thursday for the next round of biopsies and tests. I actually love going because I love the people: the nurses, the doctors, the support staff and the other transplant patients who are on the same schedule as me or whom I met in the hospital. We're kind of a clique. All the doctors in the cardiology department know me because of the rarity of my disease, even if I don't remember them. I guess they're going to write about me someday. I never knew I was so special. Please keep in touch. You are always in my heart. God bless and keep you in His care.

□

April 4

Dear Dr. Deng:

I understand from Sue that the Holter monitor was abnormal. I did not experience any irregular beats that I was aware of during the 24 hours I wore the monitor. However, I have had some since. I am concerned about it because I feel it. What are your thoughts on this? Has the giant cell come back or is this damage to my heart from the chemo? Or is this some sort of valve problem, tumor or nutritional issue? I know that my blood sugars have been very low at times. Would appreciate your feedback. God bless and thank you for your care.

☐

April 4

Dear Dee:

We are sooo happy that you are coming to see us. We're sort of on pins and needles here. The Holter monitor test came back abnormal. I'm in and out of some sort of heart block. Take your guess, from the chemo maybe? Remember, with this giant cell thing I don't have to have side effects that anyone else has had. Anyway, I don't know what they're going to do about it, if anything: meds, more tests, another pacemaker? Who knows? This new situation falls into the "never a dull moment" category.

Dee, I feel so inadequate. Writing has never been my gift. I'm like Moses, please pick somebody else. But there is a story to be told or at least written down for whoever might need to read it. It's too overwhelming sometimes, trying to envision the work as a whole; revisiting the experiences I'd like to forget. So I've been working on several chapters at the same time. Then I put it away for days at a time, only to be called back.

☐

April 5

Dear Nancy:

(Church friend, New Jersey)

Please continue to pray for us. My new heart has developed an irregular rhythm. I am in and out of what they call second-degree heart block. I don't know why. . . . In two weeks I have a consult with a specialist and will probably begin another round of tests. The doctors have cancelled my physical therapy until we find out what is going on. Thankfully, I am still allowed to walk, which I just love to do.

□

April 9

Dear Dee:

It's only 10 a.m. here and it is already 70 degrees. It snowed on Sunday! We're having March weather in April. No news yet on the blood work from yesterday, but the doctor said he does not think the heart block thing is "worrisome." We can't wait until you come. Jim wants to know if you and Craig would like to go to a Yankee game? He would!

□

April 10

Dearest Barb:

(Old friend, North Carolina)

 I feel so wonderful I can hardly stand it. I hit an all time low last week (antibiotic response) but that's over. My hair is growing back. It's real short and gray. I may never be able to color it again because of my hyper-reactive immune system, so I've learned to like it a lot! I'm still in isolation from the blood count, so Jim and I aren't out doing anything yet, but I'm a mad e-mailer. . . .

□

April 26

Dear Treasured Friends:

 The visit to New York yesterday was not surprising, but was disappointing. The doctor thinks that my heart was damaged in the preservation phase before it got to me. I'm going into NYPH/C this Wednesday for an electrophysiology study; the same test I had at St. Francis after which I coded several times. If the damage on the conduction pathway is where the doctor thinks it is, in the Bundle of His (a track of specialized heart cells through which an electric impulse must pass), I'll be admitted and they'll insert a pacemaker the next day. If he is wrong and the damage is higher up, they will discharge me and do nothing.

 I have my own theories about why this happened: chemo or return of giant cell, but it doesn't change the treatment. It does, however, affect the outcome. If the damage is from the chemo, the pacemaker will be a permanent fix and that will be the end of it. If the damage is from other possibilities, the pacemaker will be a temporary fix, as the deterioration may be progressive.

 Honestly, I would be more comfortable with the pacemaker in, as with the second-degree heart block I keep dropping beats. Though I'm not looking forward to adding to the development of my character and faith with this new (albeit repetitive) experience, I'll be glad when the week is over. Please pray for all of us and for a positive outcome. I am so excited about coming to California on May 10th and I'm going to hold on to that plan for dear life. God bless you and thank you.

☐

May 2

Dear Nancy:

So many prayers have been answered these past months. I prayed all the way through my test yesterday and felt God's presence with me. They put my heart through its paces yesterday with drugs that sped it up and slowed it down and a pacemaker that did the same thing, but they could not reproduce the problem. They felt that the pacemaker surgery was too risky for me, so close to transplant and with a low white count, particularly for a problem that may have resolved itself. The wonderful news is that they have changed their thinking and no longer believe that the heart was damaged before I got it. I can't tell you what a relief that is. . . .

We now have a little reprieve until the next round of tests in three weeks. I am so grateful for the quiet times, when the biggest issue of the day is what I am going to make for dinner.

☐

May 6

Dear Petie:

(Church friend, Long Island)

Jim and I were in church yesterday, up in the balcony by the choir, and it was wonderful to be there. My counts have not come up but New York and I have decided that they're not going to, that this is my body's response to the medications that they cannot cut. The bottom line is that I need to start getting out more, which is not to imply that I will be foolish. I will still wear a mask in public. I will not go places at high traffic times, except church. We will sit away from other people. But, we will begin to add some normalcy to our lives.

This is very freeing. New York and I are learning about this very rare disease that I have had. It appears that I cannot tolerate some of the medications I've been receiving. But we're still headed to California on Friday to visit our daughter for ten days!

□

May 20

Dearest Barb:

(Neighboring friend, New Jersey)

We just got back from California last night. We went to Santa Barbara to see Lauren and to Orange County to see our old friends. The greatest thing was that we were having such a great time it was easy to forget I've been so sick. I talked the doctors into canceling my weekly blood draws since the counts haven't come up since December. Too many ups and downs and we're not doing anything about it anyway, so why be a pincushion. It gives me a little more control over my life, at least in theory.

□

May 23

Dear Nancy:

We got some not so good news from New York yesterday. My cardiac biopsy of Tuesday came back at a high rate of rejection. They opted not to put me in the hospital for fear of my picking up a hospital based infection, and also because I look so good. A home health agency is coming in today and for the next three days to administer high doses of Prednisone.

The rejection episode is not unexpected as I've been unable to take the triple-drug transplant medication protocol since last November, because my white cell count stayed too low and the med is bone marrow toxic. The Prednisone means chipmunk cheeks, greater susceptibility to infection (in addition to immunosuppressive drugs and low white count) and the scariest of them all, emotional ups and downs. I've already warned the family that I am not responsible for anything I say or do over the next month and no pictures. The bottom line is that I have done it before so I can do it again. God has brought me this far; He's not going to quit on me now. I refuse to be beaten by results on paper!

☐

May 23

Dear Rizz:

(Church friend, Long Island)

As it turns out, we did not go to the City today. My biopsy from Tuesday came back positive for rejection. So as of yesterday afternoon we were scrambling to arrange at-home IV therapy for today, and if not I would have been admitted to the hospital. I'm here and had my first of three days of high doses of IV Prednisone. Back to chipmunk cheeks and the threat of gaining 30 pounds in a month! The nurse was really nice so we had a good visit in the midst of the treatment. We share a Dutch heritage.

☐

May 25

Dearest Dee:

I'm doing great. Face is red, eyes are puffy, but so far my emotions are in check. Couldn't ask for anything more. Even better, my own doctor is on call all weekend, which brings me great comfort; there are about twenty transplant doctors. Repeat biopsy a week from Tuesday. I don't know where they're going to go from here in terms of treatment. The doctors said I couldn't reject with so few white cells, but I guess they were wrong.

The kids and Jim take these setbacks real hard. I realized recently that they were in part taking their cues from me, so I cleaned up my act. Besides, I look and feel wonderful. Again, I think they are mixing up my paperwork with someone else's.

We're headed up to the farm today after my last treatment, if everyone in the state of New Jersey is healthy and if I feel well. I miss Ruffie (he's been at the vets with a problem of his own) and can't wait to bring him home. I've been baking all morning, my absolute favorite thing to do: banana cream pie for my brother, a chiffon cake with raspberry sauce for my mother and an eggless, butterless, dairyless applesauce cake for my sister. What a mess I made! Jim tinkers at his desk with the bills and the mail while I cook. It's a very Norman Rockwellian scene.

□

May 29

Dearest Dee:

I'm doing well. The IV Solu-Medrol put my teeth on edge and the taper dose of Prednisone isn't much better, but for some miraculous reason I started to feel great again yesterday afternoon. I am sooo grateful for healthy days. Jim and I are headed to the City tomorrow to begin the next round of testing for the arrhythmia. The repeat biopsy is Tuesday, June 4th. In the meantime, I'm working on the book.

□

June 3

Dear Dr. Deng:

I left a message for Sue this morning. I felt pretty crummy all weekend: upset stomach, low-grade headache, no fever, just not myself. Better today. Maybe related to the steroids? Do you want to see me when I come in tomorrow for the biopsy or just keep the clinic visit for Thursday the 13th?

Trying to understand this rejection thing. Since March, my heart has been irregular and I've had low-grade headaches that I attributed to swelling sinuses from spring allergies. I assumed it was a minor issue. Took Tylenol only once. Other than that, no signs.

Interesting point: my heart is less irregular since the IV Solu-Medrol. They want to repeat the Holter in two to three months. We discussed the heart block issue in relation to the rejection episode. Given 80% sensitivity of the biopsies, is that possible? They do not feel I have a conduction problem now. However, they noted that my magnesium level was low and feel that may be a contributing factor for other irregular beats.

I need your feedback regarding our upcoming anniversary party (roughly 140 people). Whether the biopsy is positive for rejection or not, should we cancel it? I never expected the white cell count to stay low this long. Now we have increased susceptibility to infection from the steroids. It is increasingly looking like a bad idea. Tell me what you think. Have a great day. God bless.

□

June 7

Dear Judy:

(Church friend, Long Island)

New York finally called yesterday. The cardiac biopsy was negative. Praise God! I was so exhausted upon receiving the news that I took a long nap and still slept well last night. Planning to have a nice quiet day at home today, given the rainy weather. It kind of gives you permission to snuggle in with a good book. Thank you for your care and concern — love those Mozart operas! God bless you.

□

June 17

Dearest Joy and Lynn:

(Professional colleagues, New Jersey)

Just a quick note to let you know I'm doing well. I walk a fine line between health and concern for some particular issue of my health. . . . My doctor is adamant that the anniversary party should go on as planned, but that I will not be allowed to kiss and hug everybody — which will be very hard for me!

□

July 20

Dear Dr. Deng:

FYI: The irregular heartbeat that disappeared after the first treatment with Solu-Medrol returned three days ago. I have no awareness of the heart block as before; just brief fluttering and what I suspect are premature ventricular contractions. I feel great, strong and healthy and vital signs are good. I am scheduled for a biopsy and clinic visit next week. As we discussed at my last visit, I think the irregular rhythm might be linked to rejection. We'll see if the biopsy picks it up. I'll bring pictures of the party. It was a beautiful day. God bless you.

July 22

Dear Linda:

Great to hear from you. I was doing really well; walking three miles at Caumsett State Park every morning and hitting golf balls at the driving range at Sunken Meadow every afternoon. Feeling very full of myself. Then I started blacking out; once last Saturday when we were out in New Jersey at my son's place and twice last Wednesday when I was alone. So when I told New York about it on Thursday, they said come right in and we've started a whole new round of tests. Now, of course, I cannot drive for fear of this happening while I am on the road, and there goes my independence and this beautiful thing I had going. Can't seem to get (and stay) in the wellness mode.

The good news is that my white cell count is coming up: 4.5!!! I've got my first cold, but we've held off on the Cipro unless I run a fever, which I haven't. The Cipro bottoms out my count and causes arrhythmias. So I don't want to take it unless I have to. Could be headed for the pacemaker that I managed to avoid back in May. That would be the end of my golf, which sounds like a small thing, but means a lot to me.

□

July 23

Dear Dr. Deng:

FYI: I'm having about 3-4 spells per day, not exactly blacking out, but feeling like I am going to. I grab on to the person I'm with to keep from falling. The feeling passes quickly with no apparent sequela. By the time I take pulse and blood pressure, everything is normal, no changes. Other than the spells, I feel great, albeit cross as my activity and independence have been restricted. I talked to the electrophysiologist yesterday. He is doing the tilt table test on Thursday and will check the Holter too. I'm headed in today to see the neurologist – re facial tics as discussed.

□

July 23

Dear Dr. Deng:

Just got a call from the test doctor. We just got back from the City where I had an appointment with the neurologist. It is confirmed that the second degree heart block is back and that we should put the pacemaker back in. I agree. The doctor also said he was going to talk to you tomorrow morning about putting me back in the hospital. Don't you think I should be? I am scheduled for an MRI of the head for Monday (to rule out neurological pathology behind tics and tremors), which I understand I would not be able to have with the pacemaker in. Quite a list of challenges to sort out. Talk to you soon I'm sure.

□

July 28

Dear Dr. Deng:

FYI: Home from the hospital yesterday afternoon, after pacemaker insertion for arrhythmia. Quite a harrowing experience. In the Recovery Room, I experienced palpitations in my chest. When I looked at the monitor, it looked like coupling of PVC's as well as isolated multifocal PVC's. I pointed it out to the nurse, who said it was generally normal after a pacemaker insertion. I knew it was not. The strip showed a p wave, followed by a long pause, then PVC followed immediately by a pacer spike and QRS complex. But by the grace of God, the electrophysiologist stopped by at 7:45 p.m. to check on me. He saw the strips, paged the surgeon and the two of them reprogrammed the pacemaker. For me, it was a flashback to last year, a heart rhythm out of control. I don't know enough about modern cardiology to even guess that the rhythm could be fixed by changing the settings on the pacemaker. . . .

□

July 31

Dearest Barb:

I just got back from New York. The doctors are now exploring the underlying cause of the arrhythmia. My doctor wants to rule out the return of the giant cell myocarditis in the new heart.

There was some discussion today over the risk of dislodging the pacemaker wires, as they have not had sufficient time to grow scar tissue to keep them in place. The biopsy instrument takes tissue samples from the same place in the atria and ventricles where the pacemaker wires are located. The doctors are always weighing risk versus greater risk in making decisions about my care. It never seems to be a case of good versus bad, just bad versus worse case scenario. I feel sorry for them sometimes. They are trying so hard to make me well. They are very clear about the fact that there is more about the aftereffects of this disease that we don't know than we do know.

It's a good thing God is in charge. It's all way too stressful for me to handle. I told Jim that I presently have so many holes in me I wouldn't be surprised if I started to leak. Anyway, the miracle is that I feel wonderful and actually look a whole lot better than when I saw you last. Despite these issues, I continue to improve. Ironic, isn't it!

☐

August 9

Dearest Barb:

Praise God, the biopsy results came back negative for both giant cell and rejection and the pacemaker is working great. I have my independence back and I can drive again!

I can't seem to reach a state of wellness where I am free of concerns, where somebody says go and enjoy. For some reason, I need to live on the edge. When the fall comes and flu season returns, I won't be able to return to normal activities as I had expected. I truly feel well enough to participate in life, but I don't think my count will allow it. I hesitate to buy tickets to a play, I don't sign up for a class, I am not active on any committees at church even though I am an elected member, we haven't been out to dinner for ages – except when we were on vacation and then only outdoors. It's as if everything is on hold. And yet, I feel wonderful, I am grateful to be alive, I appreciate the beauty of every single day and I try to give back whatever I can in my limited capacity.

At the very least, I pray frequently for lots of people. You and your mother are always on the list. That's the best thing I can do to change the world at this time. I've decided that my next career is going to be philanthropy, but I don't have any money to work with so I'm praying about that too. I still want to do something about AIDS in Africa and that will take a lot of money, so I'm asking God to have me win the lottery. After all, if my chances of getting giant cell were 1 in 40 billion, anyone with that kind of luck certainly can win a lottery where the chances are 1 in 200 million. Right?

You may find flaws in my reasoning, but my intentions are good, so I think God is listening. I've already told Him that I'm going to give it all away. How could He turn me down?

□

August 12

Dear Dr. Deng:

I had a rough night last night. Felt surprisingly/uncomfortably like one year ago: pronounced heartbeat, fitful sleep, nightmares, maybe a little short of breath, not sure. No changes in vital signs. . . . I'll be home if you want to call. I'll get a ride in if you want to see me. I don't want to go to the ER. [Found out later, this fearful episode was a reaction to my sleep medication.]

□

August 16

Dear Dr. Deng:

I remain grateful for your continually prompt responses to my e-mails, despite your busy schedule. I am feeling better, as discussed. This all remains a frightening time for me, despite my optimism, and you are a help to me that is beyond measure.

A year ago today I was a healthy person. A year ago tomorrow, I was not. As I reflect on the events of the past year, it seems to come down to an incredible piece of bad luck juxtaposed against a series of incredible blessings. To say that I have learned something from the experience is an understatement. However, I would never have chosen to learn this way. I now understand suffering. Dr. Rachel Remen says in her book that suffering builds integrity. I think suffering also opens our eyes to grace. Every minute I'm alive is a reason to be joyful. Every human interaction is important. Nothing is trivial. God's love comes to us in many forms: husbands, children, family, friends and sometimes in unexpected experiences of suffering and of pain. Which is how I was blessed with meeting you.

When I was admitted to CCU at Columbia on September 5, 2001, you were the first person I met. I remember you standing next to Jim, talking. I saw the pain on Jim's face. It hurt so much to see him in so much pain. Intuitively I knew that you cared, that I mattered to you, and this knowledge made all the difference in the world to me. I knew also that my destiny was not in your hands, that you alone could not save me. But I knew that on that journey, whatever course my illness took, you cared about me the person, not just me the patient.

Dr. Deng, there are no words that can adequately express how grateful I am to you for your care. What a blessing you have been and continue to be in my life. Thank you for being who you are, and for studying all those years to become the wonderful doctor that you are. Thank you for being in the right place at the right time and for saying the right words that gave me the strength to keep fighting. Thank you for your kindness to my family, for the time you took to make yourself available to them, to address their questions and allay their fears. Thank you from the bottom of my heart. God bless you.

□

September 30

Dearest Ro:

All positive energy received and appreciated! The final aspect of my "annual exam" is inpatient testing this Wednesday. Jim and I have to be at the hospital at 7 a.m. and I am on the OR schedule for 8 a.m.

Last week I had the outpatient tests, which included a MUGA scan to test heart function. Wednesday is the 8 a.m. cardiac cath (vessels) and a cardiac biopsy (rejection and giant cell). We should have a pretty clear picture of how I'm doing with these three test results. My white cell count is still down, but I feel great.

We are having a beautiful Long Island fall so I am again out walking my brisk three miles every day in our local state park. I'm also hitting the golf ball at a driving range several times a week. For some unknown reason, I am better at this than ever before, which is mysterious. My doctor said no to tennis so I had to cancel the round robin I had signed up for.

October 20

Dear Susan:

(Church friend, New Jersey)

Well, here is another chapter of my exciting life! Jim's mother couldn't see us this weekend because she had dinner plans for Saturday. So, because my white cell count was up, we decided to walk in Marsie's breast cancer fundraising hike at the Delaware Water Gap instead. On the Whitestone Bridge, we rear-ended the car in front of us, which had stopped suddenly, and got hit by the car behind us. The guy who caused the accident, the first car, drove off. I saw the first hit coming so I braced my legs against the floorboard and locked my knees. I didn't expect the second hit. Immediately, I felt a pain in my lower back and right hip. We suspect that Jim's car may be totaled, or maybe we'll just wish that it was as the damage was so extensive. No one else was hurt, not even Ruffie, thank God.

The ambulance took me to Jacobi Hospital in the north Bronx (not my favorite NYPH/C, but we had excellent care). Ruffie had ridden with us in the ambulance (no alternative!). At the hospital Jim asked the EMT what we could do with Ruff. The reassuring reply: "Don't worry – I'll just tell the nurses he's your seeing-eye dog. Right! Our twenty-year old blind-deaf pet a seeing-eye dog. Hysterical!

The kids had just arrived at the annual Gladstone horse event two hours away and responded to their father's call for help. Everybody felt bad. In the confusion of details and feelings of guilt, helplessness and yet another crisis, we realized at 8:30 last night, long after the kids had left, that all of my medications were left in the trunk of Lauren's car – medications that I can't live without. Jim had to drive four hours before my next dosing time to get the medicines back. Needless to say, we've decided to write it off as a bad day. . . .

☐

November 15

Dearest Friends:

Apparently I fractured a disc in my neck in the car accident; great deal of pain. Heart continues to deteriorate electrically. May pull out pacemaker and put defibrillator back in sometime in next few weeks. A stopgap measure until we find out what's behind all of this. Despite pain, feel wonderful. No failure or decompensation from a cardiac standpoint. Praise the Lord. Love you all. No trip to Philly anytime soon. God bless.

□

November 19

Dearest Susan:

Now they're not sure about the fracture. Some areas of "sclerosis" showed up on the CAT. They've scheduled a nuclear bone scan in two weeks to rule out abscess or bone cancer because the pain is not classic disc. Valium is the only thing that helps which leads me to believe it is muscular. You know how I am on Valium!!! Don't be surprised if I repeat myself and remember even less than usual. . . .

□

November 20

Dear Dr. Deng:

FYI: Woke up this morning and almost fell out of bed. Jim caught me; primarily balance, some dizziness. Something not right; something new. BP and weight okay. Neck pain increasingly better. CAT showed spots of sclerosis on spine. Scheduled for nuclear bone scan December 4th to rule out abscess and/or bone mets. He said to watch for cerebral palsy type gait or frequent urination to indicate pressure on spine from abscess. I will call him this morning and Sue when she comes in. No fever.

□

November 25

Dear Susan:

Thanks, but not feeling so strong right now. So many issues . . . thanks for your love and prayers.

☐

November 29

Dearest Gin:

(High school friend)

I have not been well these past weeks. A number of complex and seemingly unrelated medical issues have arisen. I just got out of the hospital last week. I had a small stroke (symptoms are resolved!). . . . We spent Thanksgiving with our son and daughter — and have two pieces of wonderful family news: Brad is engaged to be married to a childhood friend and Lauren was just accepted in the MBA program at Seton Hall. In the middle of the chaos of my health, unexpected blessings happen that lighten the burden. We are overjoyed for the children on both counts.

☐

December 18

Dear Everyone:

We miss you all always, but this time of year especially we long for the comfort and joy of those we hold most dear. I'm headed into the hospital tomorrow and scheduled for surgery on Friday (I've made the doctors promise I'll be home for Christmas). The heart continues to misbehave electrically so they're putting the defibrillator back in. Can't wait to get out of the hospital so I can finish my holiday baking. Anyway, God is good. As tough as this year has been, I am grateful to be alive, to be a mother, a wife and your friend. Merry Christmas. We love you with all of our hearts.

☐

January 13, 2003

Dear Gin:

I'm feeling much better since the defibrillator insertion. So much better in fact that I am amazed. I think I told you that my prayer is that the heart will heal itself electrically. I am presently not due back in the City until the week of February 3rd, which is the longest tether I've had since this whole thing started. I love all the hospital staff dearly but am grateful to have this reprieve. I'm always baking things for them, so am in the process of planning the next delectable goodie with a Valentine's Day theme.

We just celebrated Brad's engagement with a party at Mother's on Saturday night. These life events are the things that I so desperately wanted to live to see.

□

*"So I tell you, whatever you ask for in prayer,
believe that you have received it, and it will be yours." –* Mark 11:24

20 NEW YEAR'S RESOLUTION

End of December, 2002

As New Year's Eve 2002 approached, and as my e-mails show, I was not in the best of shape physically, spiritually or emotionally. Thank goodness I could speak truthfully to my friends – in the e-mails and calls – of elation one minute and near despair the next.

I had been out of the hospital for one week since re-insertion of the defibrillator. With the rejection episode in October, the neck pain (from the car accident) and the stroke in November and the ongoing heart arrhythmia, the past several months had been discouraging ones. (Understatement!!) For the first time in this whole experience, I had intractable pain and debilitating nausea. The newly prescribed immunosuppressive medication made me nauseated and gave me a headache. For several weeks I did not move off the couch. I knew from previous experience that the side effects would decrease over time, but that wasn't terribly comforting when I was in the throes of such discomfort. Elation and near despair – that's the roller-coaster way it was.

For tax purposes, Jim and I were reviewing the costs involved in my trips to the City for testing: parking, gas mileage, tolls and meals. In the first six months of 2002 I made thirteen trips in to NYPH/C. In the second six months, one or both of us made thirty-nine trips for assorted tests, visits, blood work, consultations and two hospitalizations. What a year it had been!

It was just before Christmas that the doctors re-inserted the defibrillator. The pacemaker from the previous July had not been able to fix the whole problem: runs of ventricular tachycardia began to show up. I wore an external cardiac monitoring device for most of November and December. Insertion of the new device would do nothing to prevent the underlying reason for the rhythm disturbance, but it would save me from a life-threatening arrhythmia if it occurred.

I saw myself as a failure, as a person who was failing physically as well as emotionally. The need for this device was just one step closer to another transplant. I was pretty down. After my one-year anniversary in October, it seemed everything was now going wrong.

At the same time, I was drifting. I wasn't sure God was paying attention to me. I just couldn't make sense out of what was happening to me. I kept thinking that if I just tried harder, exercised, stuck to my diet, took my medications, got plenty of rest, stayed out of public places, if I just did exactly as I was told . . .

But you see, that was the problem. I never was in control, not of my illness, not of my recovery and not of my life. I was soon to be reminded yet again that my life is completely in God's hands. How foolish of me ever to think otherwise.

On the Sunday before New Year's Eve, our pastor preached a sermon on New Year's resolutions. I had been ruminating about that exact thing for awhile. What kind of a resolution can a sick person like me have anyway? I can't work. I don't drive. What kind of a goal could I, of all people, make for the coming year? Obviously I want to be well, but that's out of my control despite my best efforts to the contrary.

Our pastor suggested that our resolution could be simply to "glorify God and all of His creation." Wonderful idea!

I turned a corner that Sunday. I started praying for God to heal my heart, to heal the rhythm disturbance that was causing me and my doctors so much angst. I thought, why not give it back to God? As people of faith, we are challenged to believe in the impossible, to have hope when it is not rational.

I read an article in Oprah's magazine, *O*, by Dr. Rachel Remen – as mentioned, one of my favorite authors. She recalled a luncheon with a group of friends, all of whom were harried by life, pressured to take care of themselves by racing off to the gym, taking mega-vitamins and eating special diets. She asked why they drove themselves to such lengths, and they replied, "If you have your health, you have everything."

I used to think that was true. Now, as a sick person, I realize that adage leaves many of us out in the cold. Dr. Remen, herself afflicted with a devastating chronic disease, rephrased the statement and said instead, "If you have life, you have everything." Thinking of the sermon and Dr. Remen's remark, I found myself grateful despite all, realizing that life on any terms is still an incredible blessing. This all made sense to me, gave me comfort and a sense of purpose in the new year.

Throughout my recovery, when I could still drive, my favorite part of the day was my daily walk in Caumsett Park, the beautiful state park on Long Island about five miles from my home. The park has a three-mile track that wanders through the trees and fields of the former Marshall Field estate. The walk took me about forty-five minutes to complete. It was my time with God. In the presence of the overwhelming beauty of nature, I prayed the Lord's Prayer as I walked.

With each phrase of the prayer, I expanded the text to include my own thoughts and concerns. As I viewed the pristine landscape before my eyes, I sang, "Thy kingdom come, Thy will be done, on earth as it is in heaven."

The phrase "Give us what we need this day" took on new meaning depending on the day. Some days my thoughts were for basic needs – to love and to be loved, peace in the world, freedom to worship, food on the table. Other days, the prayers were more specific: God, today I need for you to heal this heart, to help me cope with my medications, to help me see my life from the standpoint of opportunity and not restriction, to help me be grateful for this experience, for my illness, for my new heart, for my new life.

"Forgive us our debts, as we forgive our debtors," an important phrase. Over the course of the past sixteen months I tried to name each time that I had unwittingly transgressed. I prayed for people that I had hurt and I prayed for those who have hurt me. "Lead us not into temptation" – temptation to feel sorry for myself, to be judgmental and shortsighted, to be undisciplined in my prayer life, to hang on to old opinions, painful memories, limitations.

"Deliver us from the evil one." I have come to believe that sin is really anything that separates us from the love of God – be it low self-esteem or failure to act well or forgive. To me, The Lord's Prayer is a plea for God to free us from anything that impedes our connection to Him.

As my Caumsett walk progressed, my prayers continued. Beginning with myself, I prayed for healing, understanding, strength and courage to face the future. I prayed daily for my family, for their trials, their health, their healing, their cares and their concerns. Then I prayed for others – those in need of healing, comfort, support and direction. And finally, I prayed prayers of thanksgiving for family, churches, pastors, friends and bountiful blessings, not the least of which is the gift of my life. And, always in my mind were the doctors, nurses and many other hospital staff who gave me care well beyond the "mere medical" – a touch, a kind word, a smile of reassurance. Prayer transported me beyond my concerns for myself, to prayers of thanksgiving and healing for others. By bringing me closer to God, prayer affirmed the life within me. Renewed belief in prayer, with the comfort and hope it always brings, became my New Year's resolution.

"That you, being rooted and grounded in love, may be able to comprehend with all the saints what is the width and length and depth and height – to know the love of Christ which passes knowledge; that you may be filled with all the fullness of God." – Ephesians 3:17b-19

———— ♥ ————

21   THE GRATEFUL HEART

January 2003

There is much to be gleaned from an experience such as mine. A friend asked me several months into my recovery if I had yet come to the point of thanking God for what had happened to me. I've thought much about her question. Though on the surface the critical illness produced so much pain, the reality is that it gave me a stronger reliance on God and a closer walk with Him. I have found so much comfort in that place. My illness was both very public, as I received prayer and support from so many, and yet very private as ultimately the illness was my own.

Friends sent me a book I have come to value greatly: *A Grace Disguised*, by Gerald Sittser. "Sometimes suffering is very public and sometimes it is very private; always it is unique to us personally," he writes. "Though suffering itself is universal, each experience of suffering is unique because each person who goes through it is unique. Who the self was before the loss, what the self feels in the loss, and how the self responds to the loss makes each person's experience different from all others. That is why suffering is a solitary experience. That is why each of us must ultimately face it alone. No one can deliver us, substitute for us, or mitigate the pain for us."

He goes further to say, however, that though we experience loss alone, it does not have to isolate us; loss is a common experience that can lead to a sense of community where we find others with whom we can share a sense of community. I received literally hundreds of cards and notes from kindergarten classmates, high school friends, members of churches where we had belonged in years past and from people I didn't even know, but who had heard about my illness. I felt supported by their prayers and their concern for me. In one of my difficult times my friend Judy wrote, "If my thoughts were raindrops, you'd be soaked right now."

The famed Dutch theologian Henri Nouwen is credited with saying that only one kind of person transforms the world spiritually: someone with a grateful heart. My former pastor from our church in California sent a scripture passage from Philippians, about honoring those who "came close to death for the work of Christ." He wrote, "Candace, you have come close to death for the work of Christ, risking your life to make up for those services that we couldn't do. Though you never set sail for Africa, your heart has made the journey, and you are to be honored for that.

"How can I say it, your illness wasn't because you missed the call of Christ, your illness happened in the midst of obeying the call. It may not seem so noble but being obedient is not noble, it is merely a kind of holy ordinary. In this sense it is quite brave and noble, because people are so seldom obedient! Remember C. S. Lewis in *The Screwtape Letters*, 'God is happy when we merely attempt to walk, regardless of the outcome.' How much more is he pleased with you? What really matters is where we come out on the other side of the suffering." What a dear letter to send to me; I had thought I had somehow misinterpreted the call. These words gave me great comfort.

Throughout my hospitalizations, I recall with an appreciation that is beyond measure, I received letters from the ladies who belonged to the Circles in my church. My friend Betty wrote once a week, updating me on the progress of the African Hospitals Sheet Project. (Amazingly, we outdid our goal of one hundred sheets . . . and gathered four hundred instead! The women felt helpless at my being so sick, so poured their energies into this project – "my baby." This gesture was precious to me.)

My friend Kathleen wrote and said that when I came home, she would take care of everything – meals, housekeeping and transportation to my clinic visits in the City. She and my friend Rizz determined that my husband needed to get back to work. They stepped in, brought dinners to Jim, took over my care and supported me throughout recovery! The entire church, and especially the Presbyterian Women, followed suit. Words cannot express my gratitude for their caring.

□

For reasons that are not entirely clear to me, after the re-insertion of the defibrillator device several days before Christmas 2002, I turned a corner and started to get well. Every time I thought I was all better, that I was finally where I was before the illness, I was surprised to discover I could get even better.

Recovery is an amazing process. As my body and my spirit healed there were so many firsts, so many milestones, all duly noted and lifted up in prayers of thanksgiving. My first tennis game, my first Pilates class, my first dinner out, my first trip to the City by myself – all were new things accompanied by both fear and bravado; all were followed by a sense of newfound independence.

Obviously, a heart transplant is a truly extraordinary feat of medical science. It is still hard for me to get my mind around the concept, much less the awareness that it happened to me. Were it not for the skill and kindness of the physicians and staff, the support of my family, the prayers of my friends and the grace of God, I would not be here today; a very humbling thought. But not a place I want to dwell.

Life has returned to something akin to normal. The changes and restrictions are not visible to everyone. My closest friends and family pay careful attention still to all the nuances of my routine: medications, doctor visits, test results and any sign of irregularity – a cough, a fever, a bad day. I see the concern in their eyes.

I promised my donor family that I would try to live my life in such a way as to be worthy of their gift. A gift so amazing that it defies the imagination. Surely, there was someone else out there more deserving than I. Yet in my chest, this new heart beats with joy, overflowing with gratitude.

I do not know what the future holds for me. But truthfully, neither does anyone else about any other life. I know only that I want not to look back, but reach forward. I will seek to live the life I have been given abundantly, as God intended.

"Recovery is an amazing process. As my body and my spirit healed there were so many firsts, so many milestones, all duly noted and lifted up in prayers of thanksgiving. My first tennis game, my first Pilates class, my first dinner out, my first trip to the City by myself – all were new things accompanied by both fear and bravado; all were followed by a sense of newfound independence. . . ."

"It has been two years since you heard from me last. . . .
If you would ever like to know me, I would love to know you. . . ."

———— ❤ ————

22 THANKSGIVING 2003 – A LETTER TO MY DONOR FAMILY

Dear Donor Parents:

It has been two years since you heard from me last. There is so much I need to tell you. It is not necessary for you to write back. I cannot imagine your grief and your suffering. But if you ever would like to know me, I would love to know you.

You see, I have been taking really good care of your son's heart. I talk to him every day. I feel as if I know him. I point things out to him, the ordinary things around me in nature that continue to astonish me: the reflection of light off the harbor at sunrise, the sound a bird makes in flight, the smell of horses, the color of autumn leaves, the perfection of a strawberry, the smell of fresh bread, the taste of warm apple pie. I wake up in the middle of the night sometimes too excited to sleep, so grateful am I to be alive, with my husband and my puppy dog making sleepy sounds next to me in bed. My days begin and end with a prayer of thanks for your gift to my family and me. I ask God to bless you and your son in heaven.

I can't begin to tell you what a gift the past two years of my life have been. My family has recovered emotionally from the trauma of my illness, slowly but consistently as I recovered physically. My daughter had moved home in the spring of 2002 from California to be near me in my recovery. As she was unable to get a job she applied to graduate school. I call her "Sunshine." When she finishes school in December, she is heading back to California to live; dear friends are waiting for her there. Though I would like so much to keep her, with my being so well I must give her wings to fly. In this interim time, my son found the love of his life, or I guess I should say, fell in love with his childhood friend. They started Kindergarten together twenty-five years ago. Their wedding is next week. Thank you for giving me the chance to be there. I will think of you that day.

Sometime around the first of the New Year 2003, I turned a corner and started to return to my previous state of health. Every day I thought I was all better, and then the next day surprisingly I would be even better. I hadn't played tennis in over ten years. A friend invited me to play in her group. I came home after the first day on the court and called my husband crying and said, "You won't believe what I just did!" On every decent day (weather wise; all days are wonderful regardless of weather) I walk three miles in a local state park. I exercise two times a week, though I'm not terribly fond of it. I have a friend who takes me to hit golf balls at a driving range. I've found that I am much better at it than I ever was before. My ability to perform all of these things continues to astonish me.

Because it was necessary for me to stay out of public places for so long after the surgery, I kept myself busy doing my favorite things at home – things I had never had the chance to give a great deal of time to before when I was working full-time. My absolute favorite thing to do is cook. I made all homemade Christmas presents for my family last year: granola for my sister, trail mix for my son, bleu cheese crackers for my mother, sugared pecans for my Dad. I cooked for events at church, even though I couldn't go, and for shut-ins. It is a wonder my husband doesn't weigh three hundred pounds, because he was the beneficiary of all my experimentation. Such fun I had. I also played the piano every day. I love playing hymns. I didn't get really good at it, but I did get a little better. I also tried really hard to learn Spanish, but failed miserably at that. All in all, it was a rare opportunity to be responsible for nothing except myself. What a gift that was – I had the chance to do things I never thought I'd be able to do again.

In my first letter, I told you that I would try to be living my life in such a way as to be worthy of your gift. I am trying to live up to that pledge.

Since my recovery several months ago, I have started a new mission project in my church collecting medical supplies for volunteer church workers in Africa to care for families with HIV/AIDS. The project has been successful beyond my expectations. We will dedicate the boxes in December and ship them to Malawi before Christmas.

I speak in my community and write whenever asked on the subject of organ donation. I have a team of wonderful people who make up our speakers' panel. One special man is a live kidney donor who gave his gift of life to his sister in law, who speaks also as a two-time kidney recipient. Another member of the panel is a donor family who lost their son at the age of seventeen to a drunk driver. The final speaker on the panel is my daughter, who tells people what your gift of my life has meant to her. I wake up every day trying to discern how God might use me this day.

I've written a book, which I hope will help people who have suffered traumatic events in their lives. I had set a goal for myself of completing the manuscript by my two-year anniversary of the transplant. I've also just completed a cookbook of treasured family recipes for my children, my goal for completion being the occasion of my son's wedding next week. I'm in the last minute rush right now.

Forgive me for going on and on. I hope that you can find some solace in the fact that I have tried and continue to try to honor your gift in every way. I am truly sorry for your loss and truly grateful for your gift. I know that you did not deserve this terrible thing that happened to you, nor did I deserve your incredible gift. I don't make the rules, because if I did, I would much rather that the situation had been the other way around. Somehow the universe seems out of order when young people do not get the chance to live their lives.

My heart grieves for you. And at the same time, I am filled with awe, that in your darkest hour, you made such a courageous decision to give life. Words seem inadequate to describe my feelings. You've given me time, time to love my husband, my children and my family. What a precious gift that is. I live my life with that awareness. Thank you and God bless you.

Sincerely,

Candace Moose

Heart Transplant 10/01/01

♥

*"My heart grieves for you. And at the same time, I am
filled with awe, that in your darkest hour, you made such a courageous
decision to give life. . . ."*

"Love suffers long and is kind. Bears all things, believes all things, hopes all things, endures all things." – 1 Corinthians 13:4, 7

23 CANDY'S STORY – A SISTER'S PERSPECTIVE

I remember that just after Labor Day, 2001, Candy had been in the hospital for about ten days, where she had gotten a device called an "implantable cardioverter-defribillator," an ICD. I really didn't understand why she would need one just because she had a bad reaction to vaccines, but we all figured she'd be alright.

Mom called and asked me: "Mare, please go out and take care of Candy." She herself could not go because my father had just come home from the hospital after knee replacement surgery. At first I didn't want to go, because I was to start a new pottery class the next day and I didn't want to miss it. After I hung up, I realized my sister was profoundly more important to me than a class so off I went to take care of her, or so I thought.

She looked okay when I got there, but after dinner, she started to say she was burning up and her heart was racing. She asked us to take her pulse, but we could not find one. She told Jim to call 911 and he offered to take her to the hospital and she said no, call 911.

They responded and took her off to the hospital, and we followed. The doctors were doing to her what I suppose they do to anyone else who comes in in her condition. But Candy wasn't responding to anything they were doing, and you could see the look of desperation on their faces. Jim and I stood by helplessly. We couldn't stand by her and touch her or talk to her for we would have been in the way. Somehow they stabilized her, and put her in CCU. No one was sure she would live through the night. As she was lying there, drifting in and out, I would talk to her and pray to God that He would spare her.

The next day Candy was transferred to NYPH/C in Manhattan. I took Ruffie, her beloved part badger dog, to my parents for care and keeping.

The rest of the week was a blur of testing for her, no one really knowing what the prognosis would be. Almost every day I would pick up Mom and drive in to the hospital to visit Candy for a few hours. It was very difficult to see my sister, a vibrant, healthy woman, hooked up to dozens of monitors and IV bags and wasting away, while the doctors tried different treatments to stabilize her, much less trying to make her better.

I remember September 10, 2001, Candy's fiftieth birthday. She couldn't have flowers, balloons or candles and she didn't care about cake. I tried to make it special by making balloons out of colored paper with ribbon streamers and pasted-on pictures of her family and dog, so she would have something festive to look at.

I think I took Dad in a wheelchair, after his knee surgery, to see her for the first time. I know he was shocked and upset, because he got really quiet.

And I remember September 11, 2001. After that horrific morning they were not letting anyone into NYC for a few days. When they did, you could see the smoke from lower Manhattan for weeks, which was a frightening sight.

My routine for the next few weeks was to pick up Mom around 9, and go have lunch with Candy and leave around 3 to beat the traffic back home. My husband John and I would go in on weekends too. Some days she looked better than others, some days she was so depressed I would put my forehead to hers and tell her I knew she was going to get better. In my heart, I knew God could make her better, and I prayed it was His will to do so. However, one day I remember dropping Mom off at her house and crying all the way home. How much could one person bear? Why can't they find out what is wrong and make her well? It broke my heart to see my sister ill, depressed and confined to a hospital bed.

On September 29, Candy told us they had put her on the active transplant list. A heart transplant? Little more than a month ago nothing was wrong with the one she had. But we could see she was getting weaker physically and mentally. I guess they had exhausted their mixtures and potions. Now what? Pray that she gets a heart? Of course, but does that mean you are praying for someone else to die? Of course not, but that is what has to happen. Candy was ready. If a heart transplant was going to make her well, she was ready. It was a light at the end of the tunnel, the first one she had had in a long while.

Two days later, Candy called at 4 a.m. to say that miraculously there was a heart available. Brad, John and I rode in together, our emotions ranging from excitement to fear – excited that she had a chance of getting well, and fearful that she might die in surgery. We joked about starting up a very local adventure company, Passaic River Adventures, "take all the artifacts (river trash!) you want." We laughed to ease how nervous we all were.

We arrived in CCU to find Candy sitting up in bed with Jim by her side, everyone's emotions running high – excitement/fear, fear/excitement. The nurses were congratulating her as they prepped her for surgery, and took her away. We followed the gurney down the hall, not wanting her out of our sights, fearing it might be the last time we would see her.

Dr. Deng came in to the waiting room after surgery, and said everything went well and that Candy was in the recovery room, waiting to be transferred to a special post-transplant unit. Hours later we were allowed to see her after calling in to make sure it was okay. My sister was on some kind of special bed with tubes running everywhere, including a big one down her throat. The nurse told us to talk to her, that she could hear us. I stroked Candy's head and told her I loved her. She said "I love you too," which is pretty hard to say with a tube down your throat, but I understood her. It was overwhelming; my sister was alive and talking, hours after getting a new heart. I said silent prayers of gratitude.

It was quite an adjustment, but Candy started feeling better, and she looked better and better each day. About ten days later she was released. She hadn't been beyond a hospital room for six weeks. I can't imagine how good the outside world looked to her, the sunshine, the autumn colors, the fresh air, her dog. Thank God.

Candy was home only two days when she was faced with her first rejection. She was upset, as we all were, that she had to go back to the hospital and be admitted again. Here we go again, I thought. Please, Lord, give her a break. Fortunately she wasn't there long and got to go back to Mom and Dad's. Her story of all the subsequent trips and tests and challenges is an extraordinary one. She relied, throughout, on prayers and courage and faith and the kindness of all who cared for her.

My sister has, in fact, a special gift. She has the gift of making everyone she meets feel at ease and that they are a friend – nurses, doctors, technicians, the people that sweep the floors or bring fresh towels or deliver her meals. She would introduce them to us as her friend, oftentimes by name, and they all responded to her with a smile on their face and in their voice.

My sister has told me that the touch of a nurse, the kind concern of a doctor, the smile from an IV technician – all helped her every day in the hospital, in daylight and in the middle of the night. I am grateful for the loving care she received.

For this gift, and for so many other gifts, I love my sister with all of my heart. XXOO

– Mary Ann Castimore
Fall 2004

"Trust in the Lord . . . and He shall
give you the desires of your heart." – Psalm 37: 3, 4

— 💙 —

24 THE DESIRES OF MY HEART, FOR MY CHILDREN

Fall 2004

To my children, Brad and Lauren, and now to my new daughter-in-law Lauren Elizabeth – I offer you wisdoms I've gained through this experience of suffering. There would be no point to this event, unless there were lessons learned. God has demonstrated His power in our lives. Use your knowledge gained to live your lives in joy, trusting in His power to overcome evil with good, filled with His love, illuminating the world with your light.

First of all, rest assured that I feel blessed to have survived this trial. Remember the story in the book of Genesis about Jacob, when he wrestles with an angel? He walks away injured but blessed. That is how I feel, injured but blessed.

Do not live in fear. I know for a fact that on the deepest level, on the line between life and death, God is with us. I have mentioned hearing that courage is fear that has said its prayers. I don't believe I was ever courageous, but I do believe I was cared for. We were all strengthened by the prayers of so many. I was not afraid, but I was grief-stricken over the thought of leaving you. He has given us a second chance, a chance to learn from a very bad time how very precious time is. I have hoped to live to see Lauren married, to hold all of your children and to grow old with your father. That is my plan. God may have another. But do keep on making your own plans too. Never lose sight of the importance of every day.

Therefore, commit yourselves to living your lives abundantly. Maintain your faith. Make every thought a prayer. Meditate on all the good things in your life and remember that our time here is only temporary. Equip yourselves with faith so that you can face the trials of life, for they will surely happen. Don't let your bad times consume you. Let go of pain. Feed only the positive thoughts and emotions that enter your hearts. Study the Bible and pray. This will nourish a positive spirit, bringing you closer to the heart of God.

Be true to yourselves and kind to others, seeking justice for those less fortunate than yourselves. Remember that the first commandment is to love the Lord God with all your heart and all your mind and all your soul. Remember also as in Corinthians (1-13), that love never fails. Believe in the power of His love. Do these things and the peace that passes all understanding will be yours forever and ever. I love you. – Mom

"First of all, rest assured that I feel blessed to have survived
this trial. Remember the story in the book of Genesis about Jacob,
when he wrestles with an angel? He walks away injured but
blessed. That is how I feel, injured but blessed. . . ."

"My heart is overflowing with a good theme." – Psalm 45:1

25 EPILOGUE: THREE YEARS LATER . . .
THE OPTIMISTIC HEART

Fall 2004

I made it. I'm here. I'm healthy. Three years later, after many bumps in the road, I am finally better. I look just like everybody else, maybe even better.

My commitment to an exercise and diet program has paid off. The behavioral changes are subtle as well, but important to my well-being. I stay away from people who are visibly ill. I always carry a mask in my pocketbook in case I encounter someone who is ill. I wear a mask in the hospital when I go to the City for check-ups or when I travel. I can't go through the scanning device at airports because of the defibrillator in my chest. (Every single time, the transportation security personnel do a pat down. It's just part of the drill.) I carry thousands of dollars worth of life-saving immunosuppressive medications everywhere I go, always several days extra, just in case, because I can't live without them. I still don't remember certain things, some long term, some from short-term memory. Thankfully my husband thinks it's cute.

I do get sick at lot, respiratory infections mostly. I seem to catch everything. I seem to get the illness du jour more severely than other people and it seems to last longer. When I get sick I am down and out for a couple of weeks with multiple visits to the doctor, multiple antibiotics and asthma medications. But the beauty of it is that I get better . . . eventually. I am noticeably stronger now. Every little thing isn't a life-threatening event the way it used to be.

I am free to make some changes now. I don't feel obligated to attend every social event I am invited to, nor do I think twice about canceling at the last minute. For anything I commit to do, I always arrange for back-up. We buy lots of tickets for things that we give away. My sister and her husband saw "The Producers." My brother and his wife went to hear Eric Clapton. A new friend, an opera buff, got to hear Pavarotti's last performance at the Metropolitan Opera. We missed a wonderful wedding in Montana, one of Brad's college roommates, because the SARS epidemic made it just too risky for me to fly.

The hardest thing, of course, is when holiday gatherings get cancelled because either I am or they are sick. But my family and friends know these facts of my existence and understand.

I have shared in the joys and sorrows, achievements and defining moments in the lives of family and friends, for life has moved on. Wonderful and terrible things have happened to those that I love. A dear grammar school friend died suddenly of a heart attack. A wonderful mother of two has died of cancer. My sister has climbed more mountains and continues to be healthy herself. My brother has raced more cars. My children are happy again. My husband smiles a lot more. My family is more relaxed.

The invisible tether that connects me to the Transplant Clinic at NY Presbyterian has gotten longer, but the tie is no less strong. We communicate about everything: dental work, travel, colds, flu, test results, blood work, all the medical stuff and all the family stuff too, babies, weddings, kids and anniversaries. I now need cardiac biopsies only once every three months. My pathology reports are finally zero for rejection. The biopsy could be a frightening procedure if I let myself think about it but the truth is that I love the staff so much, I can't wait to see them!

The Transplant Program staff, both inpatient and outpatient, are still collectively and individually the finest people I have ever met and I am so grateful not only to be in their care, but to know them as people.

Dr. Deng continues to be a major influence in my life. An encounter with him is always a life-affirming event.

I still wake up every morning with a prayer, "Thank you, God, for this day. Thank you for my heart. Thank you for my life. Please bless my donor family in their grief." The grief of my donor family is never, ever far from my heart. I look at my own children and can't imagine what it would be like to have their lives ended at seventeen. I've met young people in the waiting room of the transplant unit: heart transplants and others. Kids way too young to experience so much suffering.

And I end my book with a plea. Ever in my mind is that we are the lucky ones. The few who out of so many on waiting lists, got a chance. My own story ends in joy, but so many do not. Please, register to be an organ donor. Please, talk to your family. Please, write it down. It is the gift of life.

– Candace Moose
Heart Transplant 10/01/01
October 2004

Candace was so right when she wrote, "They say that there is no grief more profound than that of parents whose child precedes them in death." A drunk driver cut my son's life short. My husband, our daughters and I made the decision to donate Paul's organs. Through donation we have been able to make some sense of such a senseless event. We have been fortunate to have met Paul's liver recipient. Peter is a wonderful person, he is like family. □ *Paul's first heartbeat was inside of me. One day I dream of hearing his heartbeat again even though it would be in someone else's chest. I would love to know what that special person has done with his life after receiving Paul's gift. I say special, because anyone who received Paul's heart must be very special; Paul was a very loving young man and had the biggest heart anyone could ever have.* □ *I dream of one day receiving a letter like the one that Candace wrote to her donor family. I want to know how my son's heart recipient is doing: How has his life changed? How has he made a difference in this world? I want to know everything about him. I also must face the fact that I might never know him and I might never get that letter. And this we accept with understanding.* □ *Thank you, Candace, for sharing your letter. When I read it I felt very excited and emotional — as if it were the letter I have been waiting for. I could feel your love and appreciation for the gift you received. I know my son's heart recipient must feel the same way, and even though he has not written I want to believe that just as you remember your donor, he remembers Paul every day and prays for him in heaven. I hope that those donor families that have not heard from the recipient of their loved one's gift will keep a copy of this letter with them, and every time they feel that profound grief they read it and find solace in it. I know that I will.* □ *Candace, you give us hope and validate that we did the right thing when we consented to donation.* — Celina Lopez, a Donor Family Member

"What I feel is most important in this concept of differing perspectives is that these perspectives all are complementary. They fit together, each sharing in telling the story of Ms Moose's experience."

❧

26 LOOKING FORWARD IN MEDICINE –
SHARED PERSPECTIVES

What is the role of the physician in this process so elegantly captured by Candace Moose? If I were, as the heart transplantation cardiologist of Candace Moose, to put my perspective on her clinical course into a standard case summary, it would resemble the following: *"Ms Candace Moose, born September 10, 1951, is a 53-year-old female with giant cell myocarditis and a history of allergic disposition. She underwent vaccination for typhoid and hepatitis A virus on August 17, 2001. Within seven days, she experienced an acute low cardiac output syndrome and wide complex tachycardia. She was admitted to Huntington Hospital, then transferred to St. Francis Hospital where a defibrillator was implanted and heart failure therapy was initiated. Within one day of discharge, she was readmitted to Huntington Hospital the day after Labor Day 2001 in low cardiac output syndrome, with systolic blood pressure levels not exceeding 60 mmHg. Therefore, she was emergently transferred to Columbia University Medical Center, where an endomyocardial biopsy established the diagnosis of giant cell myocarditis. Although Ms Moose was placed on immunosuppressive therapy including Prednisone, Hydroxychloroquine, and Cytoxan starting September 7, 2001, there was insufficient improvement.*

For this reason, Ms Moose was placed on the heart transplantation waiting list at Columbia University Medical Center [NYPH/C] on September 29, 2001. A donor heart became available on October 1, 2001, and Ms Moose underwent successful heart transplantation.

After discharge on October 11, 2001, a routine endomyocardial biopsy showed Grade III rejection according to the International Society for Heart and Lung Transplantation Classification which was treated with pulsed steroids. Neither at this time nor later on was recurrence of giant cells documented in the transplanted heart. Due to a persistently low white cell count despite early discontinuation of Cytoxan, the dose of CellCept was downtitrated. In the follow-up time, a second degree AV block, and later a nonsustained ventricular tachycardia, were documented on Holter ECG, and therefore a pacemaker was implanted in July 2002 and subsequently a defibrillator was implanted in December 2002. Additionally, the patient experienced a cerebral vascular accident in November 2002 with no residual sequelae.

The patient has since resumed an active lifestyle including golfing, tennis, and swimming. The second year annual on October 2, 2003, and the third year annual on September 29, 2004, showed normal function of the transplanted heart. At this time, the patient is having minor organ function problems from her preexisting arthritis, yet no major impairment from the transplantation medication. Her current medications include Prednisolone 5 mg po qd, Prograf 8 and 9 mg po qd, CellCept 250 mg po qd, Pravachol 5 mg po qd, Materna one tablet per day, Citracal one tablet tid, Ferrous Gluconate 325 mg po qd, Pepcid 20 mg po bid, Colace 100 mg po tid, Advair 100/50 two puffs qd, Combivent two puffs q4-6 hours prn, Senokot prn, Vagifem suppository once q week, and Tylenol 650 mg prn."

If I place the physician's summary in the perspective of this book's personal account, however, it is abundantly clear that the physician's perspective and the patient's perspective of the same situation are not at all the same. They do of course agree on routine aspects such as timing of diagnostic and therapeutic interventions, but they differ markedly in other vital aspects – such as the subjective weight or the symbolic meaning that they carry in the context of a person's own universe.

For example, while the pretransplant part of the physician's summary takes less than half of the summary's thirty-six lines, it appropriately carries far greater weight in Ms Moose's recollection of her experience. Similarly, the perspectives of Ms Moose's husband, daughter, and son differ in turn from mine as well as from hers. Further, if I were to ask Dr. Naka as Ms Moose's heart transplantation surgeon – or perhaps one of the nurses, social workers, or physical therapists mentioned in the book – for their thoughts on Ms Moose's clinical course, again their perspectives would be different.

What I feel is most important in this concept of differing perspectives is that these perspectives all are complementary. They fit together, each sharing in telling the story of Ms Moose's experience. They are, in this complementarity, irreducible in their view and number: No one perspective can replace any other. And none of the universes of the persons involved in this process can be reduced to the perspective of any other. My physician report does not capture Ms Moose's perception of the situation, for instance. Ms Moose's account report does not – and of course should not attempt to – capture the details of the physician report.

In this "shared perspectives" insight there is an important consequence for contemporary, modern, high tech medicine. Health care professionals are basically aware of the complementary perceptions of all people involved in health care situations as captured so remarkably in Ms Moose's account. And to this end, medical school and professional teaching and training must seek to implement strategies for health care professionals continuously developing this insight. Yet actually achieving this teaching goal is essential to the claim of humane practice of modern medicine. It is a vision with stunning ramifications for the healing process.

If this vision were to become routine in the daily care of our patients in all the societies of this world, several beneficial consequences could result:

☐ An increasing awareness would yield a strengthened perception of the differing roles of patients, relatives, and health care professionals in the recovery process – the role of health care professionals being those of "consultants" based on their expertise. The professionals would counsel patients and relatives about differing aspects of appropriate diagnostic and therapeutic options. The patient's role would be explicitly one of a person in charge of his or her own destiny, making the decisions for or against the specific options presented. Honoring the patient's preferences would implicitly assist in the healing process.

☐ Based on this many-options aspect of high tech modern medicine, the greater weight being placed on the patient's preferences might not necessarily coincide with the standard teachings of modern textbook medicines. This respect for preferences would influence not only the patient's perspectives in life, but also healthcare resource consumption itself: "more is not always better."

☐ The complementary perceptions of human experience in general – and of illness in particular – confirm that a patient's suffering is not eliminated merely by the physician's perspective of scientific developments. Among all health care professionals, therefore, an even greater responsibility lies in being available for moments of listening, encouraging, and connecting as two individuals sharing their concerns. "Maintaining eye contact and holding hands" are not outdated in the world of contemporary high tech modern medicine. They are a healing aspect that is more welcome, more powerful, than ever before.

– Mario C. Deng, M.D.

New York-Presbyterian Hospital/Columbia

Appendix A
Organ Donation – How You Can Help

The Journal of the American Medical Association has prepared a public service patient information sheet on Organ Donation (see page 196), and also has a website from which this information can be printed at www.jama.com. The site is very informative and covers such issues as what organs can be donated, steps to ensure donation and facts about being a donor as well as phone numbers and websites of organizations to contact for more information. In addition to organs, tissues can be donated as well such as corneas, heart valves and skin.

Donated tissues and organs may be used in people who have organ failure, who are blind or who have severe burns or serious diseases. You can specify which organs and tissues you would like to donate.

If you wish to become an organ donor, you need to make your wishes known to your family and friends. Fill out a donor card. Sign a Health Care Proxy indicating whom you trust to make medical decisions for you. Prepare a Living Will, a legal document that states your wishes in the event you become incapable of communicating. Documenting that you wish to be a donor will in no way affect your health care treatment in an emergency.

Recipients of your organs are chosen by severity of illness, time spent on a waiting list and medical factors – not by economic or celebrity status. There are no age limits for donors and there is never a charge to your family if you are an organ donor. Please, consider giving the gift of life to someone who needs it. CM

ORGAN DONATION

Organ Donation
Share life by donating your organs and tissues

Organ transplantation can be lifesaving for people with organ failure. According to the United Network for Organ Sharing (UNOS), there were more than 76 000 people waiting for organ transplants in the United States as of June 2001. Thousands of those patients may die because there are not enough donated organs to meet the demand. The main factor limiting organ donation is that less than half of the families of potential donors consent to donation.

An article in the July 4, 2001, issue of *JAMA* reports on the factors that influence families' decisions to donate the organs of a family member. The authors found that families who had discussed organ donation in the past and who had prior knowledge of the patient's wishes were much more likely to donate the patient's organs.

Type of Transplant	No. of patients Waiting for Transplant
Kidney	49252
Liver	17789
Pancreas Islet Cell	202
Kidney-Pancreas	2528
Intestine	162
Heart	4247
Heart-Lung	218
Lung	3736
Total*	76848

Source: UNOS, national patient waiting list data as of June 8, 2001.

*Some patients are waiting for more than one organ and may have registered with more than one transplant center (multiple listing); therefore, the total number of registrations is greater than the actual number of patients.

WHAT IS DONATED?

Many organs can be donated, including heart, intestines, kidneys, liver, lungs, and pancreas. Tissues that can be donated include corneas, heart valves, and skin. Donations may be used in people who have organ failure, who are blind, or who have severe burns or serious diseases. If you wish, you may specify which organs and tissues you would like to donate.

STEPS TO TAKE TO ENSURE DONATION

- Inform your family, friends, and physician that you wish be a donor
- Fill out a donor card and the back of your driver's license and keep copies with your physician, family, and attorney, and in your wallet and the glove compartment of your car
- Assign a health care proxy or a medical power of attorney, a document that indicates whom you trust to make medical decisions for you. This can be a physician, a friend, or a family member
- Prepare and sign a living will and an advance care directive—legal documents that state your wishes in the event you become incapable of communicating

SOME FACTS ABOUT BEING A DONOR

- Documenting that you are a donor will not affect your treatment in an emergency; the first emphasis is always to attempt to save your life
- Recipients of your organs are chosen by severity of illness, time spent on a waiting list, and medical factors, not by economic or celebrity status
- There are no age limits for donors
- There is never a charge to your family if you are an organ donor
- Most religions support organ donation
- Your body will *not* be disfigured (for funeral services)

Follow the steps above to be sure your wishes are followed. If you are not currently registered to be an organ and tissue donor, consider giving the gift of life to someone who needs it.

Sources: United Network for Organ Sharing, Coalition on Donation, American College of Physicians-American Society of Internal Medicine, National Institutes of Health, Health Resources and Services Administration/Department of Health and Human Services

FOR MORE INFORMATION

- United Network for Organ Sharing (UNOS)
  888/894-6361
  www.unos.org
- Coalition on Donation
  800/355-SHARE
  www.shareyourlife.org
- Health Resources and Services Administration/Department of Health and Human Services
  301/443-7577
  www.organdonor.gov
- Transplant Recipients International Organization, Inc
  800/TRIO-386
  www.trioweb.org

INFORM YOURSELF

To find this and previous JAMA Patient Pages, go to the Patient Page Index on *JAMA*'s Web site at www.jama.com. A JAMA Patient Page on organ donation was published on October 7, 1998.

Lise M. Stevens, MA, Writer

Cassio Lynm, MA, Illustrator

Richard M. Glass, MD, Editor

JAMA
THE JOURNAL OF THE AMERICAN MEDICAL ASSOCIATION
COPY FOR YOUR PATIENTS

Appendix B
Glossary of Medical Terms

Advance Directive – a document created to designate who will make healthcare decisions and stipulate what you would want done in the event you were unable to make decisions for yourself.

Angiogram or cardiac catheterization – an x-ray of the coronary arteries that is taken after injecting dye through a catheter.

Arrhythmia – an irregular heartbeat.

Atrium – the upper chamber in each half of the heart.

Autoimmune response – a physiological response of the body against itself.

Bundle branch block – a defect in the electrical or conduction system of the heart wherein there is a failure of the electrical impulse to travel down one of the main branches of the heart, resulting in the branches beating independently of each other.

Bundle of His – a track of specialized cells between the atria and ventricles of the heart through which an impulse must pass. From these the bundle divides into the right and left bundles, which go to the right and left lower chambers of the heart, causing the ventricles to beat at the same time.

Cardiac biopsy – a post-transplant diagnostic procedure whereby an instrument is passed through a catheter in the neck to the heart, from which tissue samples are removed for testing for organ rejection.

Cardiac enzymes – substances that are released into the bloodstream when cardiac damage has occurred.

Cardiomyopathy – a condition of deterioration of the heart muscle resulting in loss of function and/or electrical conductivity.

Echocardiogram – a diagnostic test of heart function utilizing sound wave technology.

ECG or EKG – an acronym for electrocardiography – a method of recording the electrical activity of the heart.

Electrophysiology study – a diagnostic test of the electrical conductivity of the heart.

Fluoroscopy – a diagnostic test utilizing a fluoroscope device whereby images are visible on a screen.

Health Care Proxy – a type of Advance Directive that stipulates a designated healthcare decision-maker in the

continued

event you are unable to make decisions for yourself.

Heart attack, or myocardial infarction – the development of the death of heart muscle tissue due usually to a lack of blood flow to the area following the blockage of a coronary artery.

Heart block – a defect in the conduction system of the heart whereby there is complete dissociation between the atria and the ventricles.

Heart failure – a condition whereby the heart fails to maintain adequate circulation of the blood.

Holter monitor – a diagnostic test of heart rhythm whereby an external box stores 24 hours of information that is transmitted through electrodes that are placed on the chest.

ICD – an acronym for an implanted therapeutic cardiac device – used to treat lethal arrhythmias – that is implanted under the skin on the chest wall, and from which wires are threaded through the veins into the heart to emit a strong electrical stimulus when the heart rate goes above a predetermined rate.

Immunosuppressants – medications that act to suppress the body's natural immune response.

Living Will – a type of Advance Directive that stipulates specifically which kinds of medical treatments you would accept or reject in certain situations.

MUGA scan – an acronym for a diagnostic test to determine how effectively the heart functions. A tracing radioisotope is injected into the bloodstream and the blood flow is scanned using a gamma camera. The scan measures the efficiency of heart muscle contractions and the size of the heart's chambers.

Myocarditis – inflammation of the cardiac muscle tissue.

Pacemaker – a device that is implanted under the skin of the chest wall with wires that run through veins to the heart, and which is set to emit an electrical stimulus when the heart rate drops below a predetermined point.

Pleural space – the space between the lungs and the chest cavity.

Perimenopausal – a term used to describe the period of time approaching menopause.

Premature ventricular contractions – a ventricular heartbeat that occurs before the normal one.

Pneumothorax – a collapsed lung.

Rejection – an episode wherein the immune system identifies the transplanted organ or tissue as a foreign invader and mounts an immunological attack against it. See autoimmune response.

Sinus node – a bundle of nerve cells located in the heart's right atrium that controls the electrical beat of the heart.

Sonogram – a diagnostic test which utilizes sound waves to form an image on a screen to visualize internal structures.

Spirometer – a therapeutic device that you breathe into as deeply as possible. After surgery it is used to encourage and measure pulmonary strength, and to expand lung volume and prevent pneumonia.

Tachyarrhythmia – a rapid and irregular beating of the heart.

Tachycardia – an abnormal rapid beating of the heart.

Titration – the dosage of intravenous medication as controlled by changing the rate of flow.

TIA – an acronym for transient ischemic attack, or a small stroke.

Vagus nerve – severed during heart transplant surgery, the vagus nerve innervates the heart causing the heart rate to slow down.

Vasopressor drugs – medications designed to elevate the blood pressure.

Ventricle – the lower chamber in each half of the heart.

Ventricular tachycardia – an abnormal rapid beating of the heart that originates from an ectopic focus in the ventricles.

❤

*"To our daughter Candace – to say that we are proud
is an understatement, but there are no words to describe
our feelings of gratitude to our Maker
for His care and keeping of you through this ordeal."*

– Emery and Lillian Castimore

❤

*" My hope is that, no matter what your belief system, you
will find comfort, strength and even humor in my story.
And know that whether you are pastor or congregant, doctor or fellow patient, friend or family member, you have the
power to heal. Every word, every gesture, every act of kindness, however small, can strengthen someone who is ill."*

– Candace Moose

Appendix C
Resources & Recommended Reading

"AIDS in Africa, a Generation at Risk." Church World Services pamphlet, undated.

"As You Go, Proclaim the Good News." *Mission Yearbook*. PCUSA (2002): 34.

Au, Wilkie. *The Enduring Heart*. New York: Paulist Press, 2000.

Bloom, Archbishop Anthony. *Beginning to Pray*. New York: Paulist Press, 1970.

Church World Service Bulletin, Spring 2002.

Cooper, M.D., Leslie T. "Giant Cell Myocarditis: Diagnosis and Treatment." *Herz* 25 (May 2000): 291-298.

Cooper, M.D., Leslie T., Ed. *Myocarditis: From Bench to Bedside*. Totowa: Humana Press, 2002.

Cooper, M.D., Leslie T., and Gerald J. Berry, M.D., Raplh Shabetai, M.D., for the Multicenter Giant Cell Myocarditis Study Group Investigators. "Idiopathic Giant-Cell Myocarditis – Natural History and Treatment." *The New England Journal of Medicine* 336 (June 1997): 1860-1866.

Cooper, M.D., Leslie T., and Gerald J.

Berry, M.D., Mona Rizeq, M.D., John S. Schroeder, M.D. "Giant Cell Myocarditis." *The Journal of Heart and Lung Transplantation* 14 (March-April 1995): 394-401.

Daniels, M.D., Paul R., and Gerald J. Berry, M.D., Henry D. Tazelaar, M.D., Leslie T. Cooper, M.D. "Giant Cell Myocarditis as a Manifestation of Drug Hypersensitivity." *Cardiovascular Pathology* 9 (September/October 2000): 287-291.

Daily Word, Silent Unity's Magazine, Ford Smith/CORBIS.

Deng, Mario C., M.D. "Cardiac Transplantation," *Heart* 2002; 87:177-184.

Edwards, M.D., Niloo M., and Donna Mancini, M.D. *The Patient's Guide to Heart Transplantation at New York-Presbyterian*. New York-Presbyterian Cardiac Transplant Program.

"Organ Donation." *Journal of American Medical Association* 286 (July 4, 2001): 124. <www.jama.com>.

Kushner, Harold S. *When Bad Things Happen to Good People*. New York:

continued

Avon Books, 1980.

Landers, John. "Shout It Out." *Transplant Chronicles* 9 (Fall 2001): 5.

Livingston, Patricia H. *Lessons of the Heart*. Notre Dame, Indiana: Ave Maria Press, 1992.

____ . *This Blessed Mess*. Notre Dame: Sorin Books, 2000.

Muggeridge, Malcolm. *Something Beautiful for God*. New York: Harper and Row Publishers, 1971.

Nouwen, Henri J. M. *The Return of the Prodigal Son*. New York: Doubleday, 1992.

Remen, M.D., Rachel Naomi. *Kitchen Table Wisdom*. New York: Riverhead Books, 1996.

____. *My Grandfather's Blessings*. New York: Riverhead Books, 2000.

Rolheiser, Ronald. *The Holy Longing*. New York: Doubleday, 1999.

Rosenstein, Elliot D., and Mark J. Zucker, Neil Kramer. "Giant Cell Myocarditis: Most Fatal of Autoimmune Diseases." *Seminars in Arthritis and Rheumatism* 30 (August 2000): 1-16.

Sittser, Gerald L. *A Grace Disguised*. Grand Rapids: Zondervan Publishing House, 1995.

Stuart, Frank P., and Michael M. Abecassis, Dixon B. Kaufman. *Organ Transplantation*. Georgetown:

Vademecum Landes Bioscience, 2000.

Tang, M.D., Wai Hong W., and James B. Young, M.D. "Myocarditis." *E-Medicine* (October 8, 2002): 1-14. <www.emedicine.com>.

The New Possibility Thinkers Bible: New King James Version. Nashville: Thomas Nelson Publishers, 1996.

The Presbyterian Hymnal. Louisville: Westminster/John Knox Press, 1990.

Winter, Miriam Therese. *The Singer and The Song*. New York: Orbis Books, 1999.

www.gcminfo.org – Patient and family centered giant cell myocarditis website with chat room.

www.litro@verizon.net – The Long Island chapter of Transplant Recipients Organization, a local support group for recipients and their families and donor families, with link to the national organization.

www.wildirisdesign.com/tso - The Transplant Support Organization; links to sites dealing with issues germane to all types of transplants.

www.mayo.edu/research/giant cell myocarditis - The Giant Cell Myocarditis Treatment Trial and Registry.